How to Get
High-Quality
Plastic Surgery...

CHEAP!

How to Get High-Quality Plastic Surgery…
CHEAP!

The Insider's Guide to the Lowest Priced,

Best Quality Plastic Surgery Available on Planet Earth!

JoAnn M. Roselli

Dreaming Awake Publications

A Division of Dreaming Awake Enterprises

Santo Domingo, Dominican Republic

Disclaimer

Dedication

This book is dedicated to my gorgeous man, who has loved me and cared for me at my worst and at my best. He has inspired me to be the best person I can be, to follow my dreams, and to leave painful memories in the past in order to forge a bright future. Thank you for helping make all my dreams come true!

Life shrinks and expands in proportion to one's courage.

~Anaís Nin

One's courage shrinks in proportion to how much one has expanded.

~ JoAnn Roselli

Foreword

Dear Friend and Kindred Spirit:

I would like to personally thank you for purchasing this book!

It is my dearest hope that using the information that follows, you are able to enjoy the kind of affordable and high-quality cosmetic surgery that I was lucky enough to find.

While the original version of this book focused only on the superb, low cost plastic surgery in the available in the Dominican Republic, in this expanded version I have included some additional information regarding other places where you will find affordable prices for plastic surgery.

I would like to make a special point of letting you know that at the time of the writing of this book, I do not work for any plastic surgeon, nor have I accepted any payment or discount from any surgeon or surgical society.

All mention of specific surgeons, facilities and associates are the result of my own research and none have paid for inclusion in this publication.

The information in the following pages I have gathered from family, friends, the Internet, and a few surgeons who have kindly granted me interviews.

This compilation is for your benefit, not simply to further the practices of international plastic surgeons. My purpose is to reach out and let people know about the great surgery and great prices available to you if you have the desire, ability and adventurous spirit to take advantage of it.

This book is in its fourth incarnation, having undergone frequent update, expansion and a few name changes.

As the field of plastic and cosmetic surgery is ever changing and growing in popularity, I have found that frequent updates are necessary.

Therefore, I encourage those with internet connection to visit my web site at **http://www.cheap-plastic-surgery.com** and sign up for my free newsletter to keep abreast (pardon the pun) of the latest updates.

TABLE OF CONTENTS

Procedure Details…What You Can Expect Before, During and After Surgery 102

Bariatric Surgery 136

…And Don't Forget to Bring Your Toothbrush! (Things to Bring for Your Cosmetic Surgery Trip to the Dominican Republic) 147

Use Your (Recovery) Time Wisely 152

A Little Advice on "After-Care" 157

One Last Word About Dominican Plastic Surgeons (the Inside Scoop) 160

Dominican Republic Travel FAQ's 169

Other Money-Saving Surgery Options 180

Introduction

In writing this book, I am surprised to find that it has stirred up a lot of emotional memories for me. I came to the Dominican Republic in the summer of 2001 for the purpose of undergoing cosmetic surgery, and I instantly fell in love with this beautiful country and its wonderful people.

Having had such a positive experience on my first visit, I returned in the Spring of 2002 with the purpose of indulging in a few more of the low cost, high quality cosmetic surgery procedures, the likes of which I would not be able to afford in the United States (my then-home).

Again, my experience was fantastic. It was at that time that I decided that I would take a chance on the Dominican Republic and make it my home. With my husband (who was born in the Dominican Republic but had spent the last 22 years in the States), our then 7-year-old son and my mother, we packed up everything we could, gave the rest away and started our journey.

Nearly 3 and 1/2 years later I am proud to say that making that move was one of the best decisions I have ever made and I wouldn't change a thing. My quality of life has improved dramatically and I am ever in awe of the amazing sights, sounds and people that I encounter every day. The transition has not always been easy, but I am certainly a better and happier person for having made the change. Here I am able to live my dream of living in a house by the beach with a gorgeous view of the Caribbean from my patio where I write. I can afford to send my son to an international school where he is learning three languages and is getting a far better education than the one I got. We are able to afford a housekeeper, who is a wonderful person and an absolute gift from above for me! All of this costs us about 1/3 of what it would have cost us in the United States.

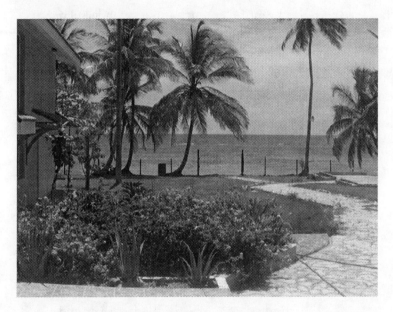

View from my patio...Hemingway eat your heart out!

After my first surgery, a tummy tuck and liposuction, I was so grateful for having found the option of having such low-cost cosmetic surgery, performed by such a highly qualified and skillful surgeon, I was moved to try to find a way to help others who would benefit from my "discovery". I knew many people in America and elsewhere were in the same situation as I...desperately wanting and needing cosmetic surgery procedures but financially unable to afford the exorbitant prices in the US and various other countries.

I was so grateful for the fact that, since my husband had many wonderful family members and friends in the Dominican Republic, I had a lot of support, reassurance, "inside information" and guiding hands to make the experience easy for me. How lucky I felt! 'Everyone should be able to have this available to them!' I thought. This book was born from that intention.

In reaching out to others who were searching for great surgery at affordable prices, I placed several postings on Internet message boards telling of my happy discovery. I received an overwhelming response from people asking for names and telephone numbers of qualified, skilled Dominican plastic surgeons as well as details of my own personal experience with having cosmetic surgery in the Dominican Republic.

Because I couldn't keep up with the number of emails I was receiving, all of them asking for more information, I decided to write this book so that I could help every interested person to get the information that they wanted and needed. In the process, I have made many new friends. That is a benefit that I didn't expect and I treasure the most out of this entire experience.

The way that total strangers can share their thoughts, feelings and helpful information is what makes the Internet the greatest invention the world has ever known!

In fact, 8 years ago I met my soulmate via the Internet (but that story is material for an entirely different book!) It is because of this man, my gorgeous Arturo that I discovered the great, affordable plastic surgery options of the Dominican Republic that I can now pass along to you.

In this, the story of my personal experience of having plastic surgery in the Dominican Republic, I will impart to you everything that I endured before, during and since those surgeries and why I am such a proponent and good will ambassador for the plastic surgeons of the Dominican Republic.

Exciting News About "How to Get High-Quality Plastic Surgery...CHEAP!"

Over the past few years since I put out the first edition of **"How to Get High-Quality Plastic Surgery... CHEAP!"** I've had numerous requests for help from my readers to arrange their travel, accommodations and other details to help them get their surgery here in the Dominican Republic. For a long time, due to my location and personal commitments, I was unable to help to the extent that I had wanted.

Recently, all of the pieces of the puzzle have fallen in to place. I discovered the perfect brand new plastic surgery clinic, PlastiCenter in Santo Domingo, and my family and I have relocated to the beautiful resort town of Juan Dolio, just a short drive to Las Americas Airport, as well as the metropolitan center of Santo Domingo.

The clinic is absolutely gorgeous...we're talking Beverly Hills standards. I am thrilled to be able to offer my clients such an elegant facility. Even though I was quite impressed with the clinics I had visited and had surgery in prior, **PlastiCenter** certainly was reigned supreme.

I was really pleased when I saw all the care the doctors had put into making the rooms ultra-safe and comfortable for their patients, including pulse-oximeter equipment in each room to monitor the patients' vital signs, inflatable leg massaging devices for the prevention of deep venous thrombosis following surgery, handrails and personal showering devices next to the toilets, safety deposit boxes for personal valuables, walkers (for those of us too stoic/independent/stubborn to call the nurse for help getting to the bathroom), and comfortable sofa/daybeds for spouses to spend the night at the patient's bedside.

There are lots of other amenities too numerous to mention here. Just rest assured that indeed I believe that they really have gone the extra 100 miles to make sure their patients get the best care in the most comfortable surroundings imaginable.

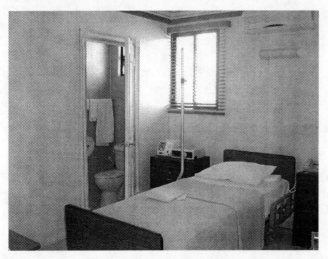

Comfy patient room with bathroom REAL close to your bed! Very important!

Dr. Guerrero, as I learned, is not only an accomplished and skillful surgeon, but is also is a high-ranking officer in the Dominican Armed Services, a pilot and a musician who plays base guitar and loves to sit in with local meringue bands when he has the opportunity and time.

On top of all that, he is such a friendly, personable and compassionate guy with a fantastic sense of humor. He kept us laughing throughout the day. I had the fortune to meet quite a few of his patients, all of whom praised him as a great surgeon and a great man.

Even though he is such an accomplished man and respected surgeon, Dr. Guerrero treats everyone he encounters with respect and puts people at ease immediately. I was struck by the fact that every time I went to his office that week, his waiting area was full of people who smiled, chatted and joked...even though most were complete strangers to each other. It was such a stark contrast to the doctors' waiting rooms I had been in (especially in the States), where people sit with their noses buried in magazines, never daring to even look up at the people around them, so quiet and uncomfortable.

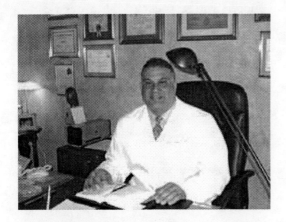

Dr. Roberto Guerrero

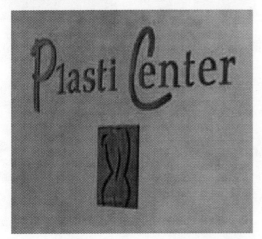

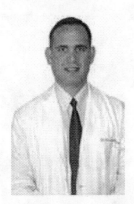

Dr. Alejandro Hernandez

PlastiCenter felt more like a little party or a get-together than the usual somber medical office…just a lot of happy, like-minded people, there to see the men that were going to help them look and feel their best. In fact, it was easy to imagine a ratings-winning reality show in the making! So, we're even working on putting together season one of **La Simetria Plastic Surgery Vacation, the Reality Show**. Dr. Guerrero definitely has star-quality. My visits to his clinic were far more entertaining than anything I've seen on TV in years! Who knows, you may be tuning in sometime next year!

I'm really excited to be able to offer so much luxury, safety, excellent medical and surgical care, great food, and wide assortment of my favorite self-improvement and health improvement learning materials to my readers and guests! It's been a long time coming, and now the time is perfect.

If you are interested in having me and La Simetria host you for your plastic surgery vacation, please contact me by email at vacation@cheap-plastic-surgery.com. If your more of a phone-talker, please contact me by telephone locally in the New York area at (718) 701-5211 or toll-free nationwide at (877) 274-0573.

(Cheap) Cosmetic Surgery Options

A recent statistic showed that 11.5 million cosmetic surgery procedures (including non-invasive procedures) were performed in America in 2005 alone. If that many people in America actually HAD the surgery, then it is safe to say that at least 50 times that amount considered having surgery but did not due to financial reasons. Needless to say, cosmetic surgery is considered a viable option by more than just movie stars and the super-rich. In fact, over $12 billion dollars was spent on cosmetic surgical and noninvasive procedures in total!

However, prices in the United States for medical care of any kind are far too high for the average American, without going serious debt. The reasons behind this are of crisis proportion. Most Americans don't have even the most basic health insurance. How is it that so many people could afford cosmetic surgery last year? There are many companies now financing cosmetic surgery, and reaping hefty returns on their investments.

So the new boobies you get next month you will continue paying for (and thusly over-paying) just like the washing machine in the basement or the Toyota parked in your driveway. By the time you figure in financing charges and interest, you will pay far more than the price your doctor originally quoted you. In many cases, patients who chose to finance their surgery will pay 3-5 times as much as the original cost. As of now, though, at least there's no fear of repossession for non-payment!

Plastic surgery financing has been the answer to many prayers. After all, we Americans are careless enough to put pizza and chicken wings on our credit cards…why not use your credit for something that will improve the way you look and feel? I have nothing against plastic surgery financing, as long as the individual goes into it clearly knowing the terms of the financing agreement and can afford the monthly payments without problems.

What about those of us who have "maxed out" our credit or don't want another bill to pay every month? Where do we turn? Are there any options other than borrowing from our retirement accounts or begging our parents for an advance on our inheritance?

The good news is that you do have options! The bad news is that your options, although affordable to most, may be less convenient and may take more of an "adventurous spirit" than what you normally would associate with a visit to the local plastic surgeon.

Simply visiting a foreign country is scary for a lot of people (myself included, once upon a time). And of course, going under the knife for any reason takes a lot of courage to begin with!

Most of us are squeamish at the thought of a needle being poked into our flesh, much less being cut, stretched, sucked and stitched. Combine the two, and you have a real exercise in *character building*.

As I mentioned earlier, having surgery in the Dominican Republic was easier for me than it would be for a lot of Americans. This was because my husband was born here in the Dominican Republic and has lots of family and friends who not only live in the DR, but also have had cosmetic surgery and are familiar with the process, the facilities and the doctors.

I had a hand to hold on to (several actually), my own interpreter and a comfortable place to stay. I had reassurance from many trustworthy sources. But the average American hasn't had such luxuries.

While the phenomenon of medical tourism is picking up steam, the unfortunate situation is that the mainstream media have a tendency to focus on the cons, rather than the pros. For more on this subject, please see the chapter, **"Globalization and You"**.

I have made it my mission to change that situation, both by sharing my story as well as partnering with a world class resort to cater to the plastic surgery tourists needing guidance, care and comfort to make the overseas plastic surgery experience a complete success.

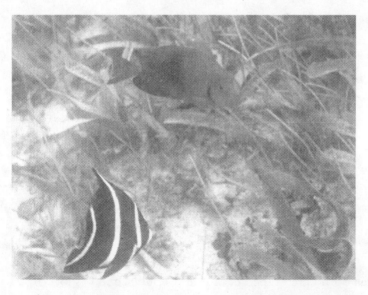

Some "friends" I made while snorkeling in my backyard.

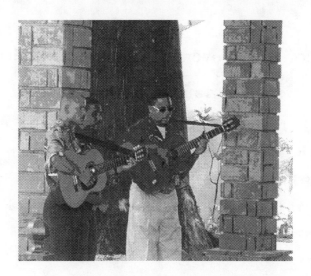

There's Always Music in the Air

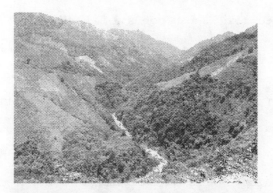

Breathtaking View of Dominican Mountain Range

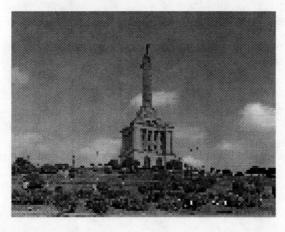

Majestic National Monument in Santiago, Dominican Republic

My Personal Discovery of Cheap Cosmetic Surgery in the Dominican Republic

Back when we first met, my husband told me that his cousin from the Dominican Republic was as big as me or bigger, had liposuction 8 years ago and now has a great body! She never gained the weight back. And in the Dominican Republic liposuction is cheap! Most everybody who has a middle class income can afford it.

Wow! I had never even really considered liposuction as an option for me. I had always been told, "liposuction is not a method of weight loss". And I thought, like I said before, only rich people could afford something like that. Not to mention all the guilt I associated with it…like only really conceited, vain people would have surgery to make them look better. It seemed so extreme, so selfish and unrealistic.

Considering myself to be an average person, I had always accepted that I'd have to live with my physical imperfections and just accept my plight. I rarely let myself consider how badly my weight problem had held me back and excluded me from certain successes I may have otherwise enjoyed.

I was picked on for being fat since I was in the 3rd grade. It seemed that no matter how smart I was, how sweet I was, how quiet I was, people would still say mean and degrading things to me. I wanted to become invisible, but year after year I just became more visible.

I literally had bullies follow me home from school, pulling my hair and throwing spit wads at me the whole way. The adults said, "She'd be so pretty if she wasn't so fat!" They thought they were complementing me with that!

When I would cry about some new insult, my family would tell me I was "too sensitive".

When I would tell the teacher that the boys were picking on me and calling me "fatso", the teacher would say, "Boys will be boys!"

I never dated, didn't go to the prom, and basically thought of myself as unlovable. I had plenty of friends to party with, but never a boyfriend. I felt so bad about myself that I never thought anyone could like me "that way".

I dropped out of college three times before I finally got my degree. Each time was provoked by my own feelings of inadequacy and generally feeling embarrassed about my appearance. I just didn't even want to be part of anything or go to class for fear of being picked on or humiliated because I wasn't 'perfect'. As embarrassing as it is to admit, I didn't even have my first real relationship until I was 27 years old!

In all those years, I was constantly dieting, exercising for hours until I would nearly collapse, trying every diet they could come up with, taking diet pills and getting nowhere.

I would gain and lose the same 40 lbs. year after year after year. It was like some Greek myth. I felt like I was doomed…like rolling a boulder up a mountain just to have it roll right down the other side. What would life be like to finally not have to feel guilty for everything I ate that didn't resemble vegetation? To get rid of fat and have it never come back! Yippee! To actually get to enjoy a holiday feast without shame and guilt? Sheer bliss!

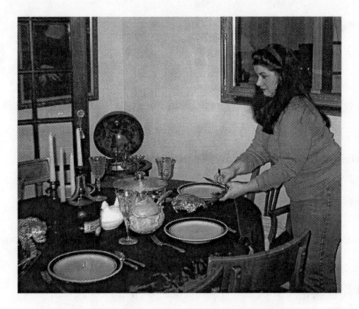

Holiday feasts were my shameful pleasures

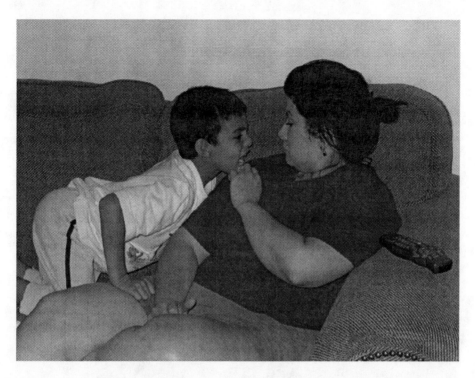

Wow, I looked even worse than I felt…and I felt horrible.

During all those years of being fat and hating the way I looked, I forbade anyone from taking my picture. Most of those photos that I wasn't able to prevent, I eventually tracked down, confiscated and destroyed.

Never did I imagine that one day I would be sorry that I didn't have any more 'fat pictures' to show the world! Alas, though the images are few and don't even reflect me at my absolute largest I think you can see that I was in dire need of the extensive surgery that I eventually would undergo.

In Search of Surgical Solutions

On a day of total self-hatred in the summer of 1998, I decided I could not go on like I had been all my life. It was just too hard. I finally had this man whom I adored. I just wanted to finally be "normal", somebody he could be proud to have on his arm.

I decided to look into having liposuction in Manhattan. I found a web site that talked about a doctor on the Upper West Side and the before and after pictures were astounding.

I called his office and they ran a credit check and excitedly informed me that I "qualified" for financing…$300.00 a month for the next 6 years, plus any financing charges! Not knowing any better at the time, and being nearly suicidal, I enthusiastically scheduled an appointment.

When I got there, I was horrified to see a giant statue of a big, fat, ugly TROLL in the waiting room! I could not believe my eyes!

Then when I met the doctor, I understood completely. It was almost an exact replica of the doctor! I mean…Physician heal thyself! None of this was giving me good vibes, to say the least.

When it was time for my consultation, I went in his office (dragging my husband with me for fear of being alone with this guy) and oddly there was some lady sitting in the office already. He didn't even introduce her as another doctor or anything! Feeling stupid and awkward already, he told me to drop my pants! I could have died.

Sheepishly, I did as I was told, at which point he said to me, "Well, I'll never be able to make you a skinny-minnie but I can probably take off about 2-4 lbs. You'll have to be in the hospital for a day or two. We'll have to roll you over during the operation. It will probably take about 5 hours. My fee is $6,000.00. The anesthesiologist and hospital will bill you separately."

And this guy wasn't even a "real" plastic surgeon. He was just a dermatologist!

Oh my GOD! I wanted to die. I was so humiliated, degraded and disappointed. I sobbed all the way home. My poor husband didn't know what to say to me. He made a lot of troll jokes, which made me laugh a little in between crying fits. I really thought I was hopeless.

Over the next few years, I continued on my diet rollercoaster. I tried the high-protein/no carbohydrate diet and lost 32 lbs. in 6 months. I felt great! Within a year, I gained it all back plus an extra 5 lbs.

We moved to Florida, I joined a gym and started working out for 2 hours a day. I stopped eating solid food and only drank whey protein. I lost 8 lbs. in 2 months of this. Then my mother came to visit, I started eating regular food again and gained it all back within 3 weeks.

There Are No Problems…Only Solutions!

In August 2001, we finally got the chance to get the surgery I needed. We came to the Dominican Republic, spent one day visiting with his family (most of whom I had never even met before), and the next day I went to Santo Domingo to meet with a plastic surgeon. To my shock, he scheduled me for the very next day!

Because I had gained and lost so much weight over my lifetime my skin had become flaccid, so the doctor recommended a tummy tuck and liposuction. I have to be honest with you…I was terrified!

I had never had any kind of surgery, and I had only been to a doctor about 4 times in my entire life. I had never even had an IV before!

It was scary and emotional, but my doctor was very, very reassuring. His gentle nature and obvious concern for my overall health and comfort level really eased me through the whole thing.

I was very impressed by the beautiful décor of the clinic and degree of professionalism of the entire staff. I really had no idea what to expect before I came to Santo Domingo, since the Dominican Republic is a small country and often referred to as "third world"…whatever that means.

In fact, as our plane touched down on the runway, we had a rather bumpy landing and my husband leaned over to me and said, "I forgot to tell you, the runway isn't paved here!" I squealed out loud in shock…but of course, this was another one of his "jokes"!

The hospital, clinic and doctor's office far surpassed those I had encountered in New York! As a lover of interior decorating, I was astounded by the marble terrazzo flooring, mahogany woodwork, beautiful original artworks, and coordinated draperies and upholstery I admired everywhere I looked.

Even though I had no idea what the doctors and facilities would be like before I embarked on my journey, I just knew I had to do it. I had to take a chance. I couldn't face another 40 or 50 years of struggling with my weight problem and most certainly not living the life of my dreams. I was about a week away from attaching a Water-Pik to my vacuum cleaner and inventing the first home liposuction kit!

I remember one of the things that impressed me most was when I got my blood taken as part of my initial medical clearance. My entire life, anytime I had to get my blood taken, the person taking it had to jab me several times before finding my vein! Ouch! It was always an ordeal. I tried to give blood once, and they ended up mangling my arm and even took a chunk out!

Well, the lady who took my blood in the clinic in Santo Domingo was so skillful; she had it done before I even realized it! I never even felt a thing.

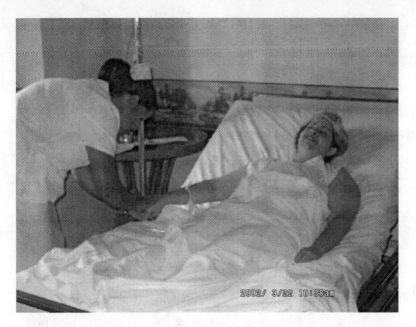

Getting My IV Inserted By A Skilled Professional. Yes, I'm Really Smiling!

Going into surgery was pretty freaky for me. Like I told you earlier, I had never even been in a hospital bed before. I cried a little out of nervousness, but then they gave me a sedative and the rest was an intriguing journey to the center of my brain.

I'm not sure what they gave me, but I came out of it feeling like I had the best trip ever…like I had just relived every pleasant moment I had ever had in my life in just a couple of hours! I had never tried any "hard drugs" in the partying days of my misspent youth, but I think I learned that day what the big attraction is.

My biggest surprise was waking up after surgery and feeling my stomach. Where did I go? It was flat as a board. No matter how much weight I ever lost, it never looked like that! I was all bandaged up and I still could tell the difference! I was psyched!

Then came time for me to get out of bed. Yikes! It hurt like hell! I felt like I had done 250 sit-ups. With all the torturous exercise I had done to myself over the years in effort to lose 50 lbs. in a week, I knew the feeling but this was EXTREME. And I couldn't stand up all the way!

It was so weird I had to laugh despite the pain! I was all hunched over and bent like an "L". As I walked, I started to straighten up a little, and within a day I was almost walking upright again.

I stayed in the clinic for 2 days, and then went to stay the house of a relative of my husband. The doctor was even nice enough to give us a ride…45 minutes away!

During the two weeks that I stayed there, the doctor came to see me three times (can you believe it? House calls!).

The most painful part of my recovery was coughing, laughing and getting out of bed. I really hated that I couldn't wash my hair for two weeks. I had to wear a compression garment that went from my knees to above my waist. Mine had suspenders and zippers down the sides. My favorite part (grossly) was that I had an accordion-like drain that sucked the fluid out of my abdomen.

Now, don't think I'm twisted…but every day I could see more liquefied fat coming out! It was amazing! I almost cried when the doctor took it out 10 days later…I wanted to keep it!

I had to have help getting in and out of bed for 2 weeks. The bed I was sleeping in was especially low. If I had to do it again, I would have had my husband put blocks under the bed to raise the height.

I didn't feel like moving around much for about a week, but then I did get out and walk a bit and go for brief car rides. The doctor came to take my stitches out within a week of my surgery. I took Voltaren for about 2 weeks, along with Advil for the pain.

I also had liposuction on my thighs and hips. I had a lot of bruising there (really ugly for about 3 weeks). I had some swelling but kept it down by taking Arnica Montana, an herbal supplement that is great for any kind of physical trauma. I had some tingling and itching as my tissues healed, but I didn't notice it all that much.

My feet swelled up quite badly, which could have been due to the tropical weather…it was the height of Caribbean summer and it was hot, baby! Keeping my feet elevated above my heart helped a lot.

The house we were staying in didn't have AC, another thing I should have considered but didn't. Yet another mistake I made…no mosquito net. Since I had to leave the windows open to let the cool Caribbean breezes waft through, the mosquitoes had carte blanche. They really chewed on me, and it was hell not being able to reach my ankles to scratch!

My advice to you: make sure where ever you stay has air conditioning.

I couldn't roll over in bed for more than 3 weeks. That was hard to get used to, especially since I am a stomach sleeper.

Another thing that was difficult to deal with was the fact that I was not supposed to take a shower for six weeks! Sponge baths only was the rule. I complied for as long as I could, but I have to admit that I caved after about four weeks and took a shower with my compression garment on, and then dried it with my hair dryer (with me in it)!

I do not encourage anyone else to do this! I shouldn't have and I risked infection by doing it. Please don't be as rebellious as I am…it usually gets me into trouble! Luckily, it didn't that time.

On the plane ride home from Santo Domingo, I had the coolest experience. It was just like something off a TV commercial. The flight attendant was having a conversation with the passenger next to me. She asked him a little bit about Santo Domingo, and surprisingly the conversation took a turn to plastic surgeons!

She said that a lot of passengers she encountered were going to Santo Domingo for cosmetic surgery, and they told her the doctors there were excellent. She mentioned that she was thinking of having a facelift and was trying to find out the name of a good doctor.

I excitedly reached in my purse and pulled out my surgeon's calling card. "I'm sorry, but I couldn't help but overhear that you're looking for a good doctor…" I handed her the card and felt good about being able to help. It was truly a cosmic cosmetic surgery moment.

The leg of our return trip from Miami to Tampa was a bit much. Being the bullhead that I am, I refused to indulge in a wheelchair and had to plod through the Miami Airport in pain. Then when we had an unexpected 5-hour delay, I broke down in tears.

This public display of emotion paid off in spades…the airline happily "squeezed" us on a commuter flight and got us home and out of the line of 210 people who were going to have to wait 5 hours to get to their destinations.

My results? I am thrilled! My stomach is always flat as a board, even at times when I used to get bloated (ladies, you know what I mean). I never have to suck in my tummy, even in a bathing suit! Hooray!!

The Second Time Around

In March of 2002, I went back for more! I wanted to get all over liposculpture, an arm lift (to get rid of the saggy "batwings") and eyelid lift. The eyelid lift was actually something I had not totally planned on, but I asked for it at the last minute and my doctor agreed.

I never liked the fatty hoods over my eyes, and had noticed that I was developing a crease in the side of my forehead because I was constantly raising my eyebrows to get a full field of vision! I had constant tension headaches because of it, too.

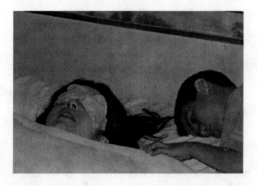

Eyes Bandaged...My Curious Son Sneaks a Peek!

The arm lift was a bit more difficult to deal with than I had anticipated. The underarms are cut in a T-shape with the top of the T being right in the crease of the armpit. The drains exited my arms near the elbows and dripped fluid constantly for about 5 days. It was really uncomfortable to not be able to move my arms, and the compression garment really irritated me. It was so tight that it made my hands swell up too much, so again like the rebel that I am, I took it off too early.

Because of my hard-headedness, my scars turned out to be wider than they should be. They have faded quite a bit over the past year, but I still regret not following doctor's orders. The scars are long and difficult to disguise for a long time. Of course, if you live in a cool climate, it is easy to disguise them under long sleeves during a good part of the year.

I am happy that my shirts fit better now. Before my surgery, I could not find short sleeves that didn't cut into my arms, and long sleeves were always tight and unsightly. I had to buy shirts that were way too big for me in order to disguise my arms. For me, the trade off for the scars was worth it but I would not recommend arm lift surgery to anyone unless they had really big, saggy upper arms.

The liposculpture really improved my figure! I had rolls of fat on my back that I really hated, and my bra always cut into me and made me very uncomfortable. Now I have a nice, smooth back, waist and hips. I had a lot of drainage from my back. I had to sleep on a plastic trash bag for about 5 days. I strapped a bath towel around my waist, as I had two drains coming out of my lower back (my husband called them my "mufflers"…ha ha ha).

If I had to do it again (which luckily I don't) I would have brought a box of maxi pads with me and taped them over my drains! It sounds queer, but it would have worked better and been much more comfortable than the methods I used. Live and learn.

My thighs are smaller, but I still need some more liposuction and maybe a thigh lift to tighten the skin up. I am wary of the thigh lift procedure, because the arm lift was so uncomfortable; I imagine the thigh lift would be much worse. Using the bathroom must be beyond difficult. The eyelid lift was a little frightening, but the outcome was very good.

I no longer have to raise my eyebrows to see well, and I have no more tension headaches! Having stitches in your eyelids is no walk in the park, but depending on how saggy your eyelids are before your surgery, it can make a world of improvement in your appearance. I had to keep tape on my eyelids for a few days, which I hated.

The bruising was minimal and really just looked like I had purple eye shadow on. I wore sunglasses all the time when we went out, even at night in restaurants. Everyone around us found me "very intriguing"…I felt a bit like a diva!

If I had to do it all over again, I would have had my husband tell the waiter we needed a table in the back because I was a soap opera star who needed to protect her anonymity from my legions of adoring fans. I believe the key to taking the edge off any difficult situation is using your imagination to put a silly spin on it. It sure makes things more fun!

Third Time's the Charm!

Most recently in September 2003, I went in for some more liposuction. I gained back a little weight, so I was up to a size 14...that was pretty much my body's favorite "set–point weight". My shape was still quite nice, but I felt too big all over. So this time I went to a different doctor, who was again recommended to me by my husband's aunt as being able to remove larger amounts of fat in one "sweep" than a lot of doctors do.

Even though I thought I was an old pro at this point, I had no idea what I was in for! Again, I found the doctor to be such a professional. He took a lot of time to explain the procedure to me and my husband, advising me on what he could do and how it would be done. I felt really good about that, because the first doctor I went to (although he was a really sweet guy and a good surgeon) didn't spend a whole lot of time advising me.

Everyone on the staff was so wonderful! They really made the whole experience a pleasure. From the lab technician to the cardiologist to the anesthesiologist and everyone I encountered in between. They were just so personable and sweet. Most everyone spoke English well, which helped make me feel more comfortable, too!

I went for my first consultation on a Monday, went back Tuesday and had my blood taken and got my cardiology consult and EKG, and was being prepped for surgery bright and early Wednesday morning at 7:30 a.m.! I've had to wait longer at the McDonald's drive through window!

The anesthesiologist was such a sweetheart. He was very reassuring, as he told me that my surgery was going to go very well and that I had a great doctor.

He also told me he was going to give me a "special blend" of anesthesia, of which he had two varieties...the one that makes you dream of Brad Pitt and one that makes you dream of Tom Cruise! I laughed right out loud. He really caught me off guard with that one! He said he was giving me the "Tom Cruise". I wasn't all that much of a Tom Cruise fan before my surgery, but I have to admit I watched "Vanilla Sky" recently and he captured my attention like never before! Hmmmm...interesting, don't you think?

The next thing I knew, the doctor was walking in the door carrying a digital camera. I was still a little out of it, but I could tell things had gone well by the smile on his face. He was proud to show me the picture that he took of the two giant beakers of fat he just sucked out of me! It was the most beautiful, disgusting picture I'd ever seen! I was thrilled! I knew what a huge difference it was going to make in my figure and in my life.

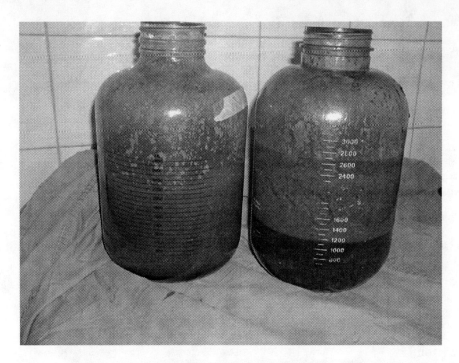

So this is what was making me so miserable for 20 years? Good Grief!

The next morning, I was a little sore but I felt really great! I got myself out of bed, brushed my hair and teeth, washed up as much as I could and slapped on some make-up. I even got dressed by myself! The nurse came in to bring me my pain meds and was shocked to see me up and about on my own.

When I got home, my butt was pretty sore, so I spent the better part of 4 days in bed. When I went in for my 1-week follow up, I was down only 1 lb. But I didn't fret about it, since I knew from experience that people usually gain weight from the post-op swelling that occurs.

After that, I shrank more and more each day. It was astounding! I could literally feel myself getting smaller and smaller. I stayed in loose, baggy clothing for the first 3 weeks so it was hard to see the difference but I could feel it.

When I finally got my nerve up to try on some jeans (which were too small for me to wear comfortably before my surgery), I was scared. I knew I would be really depressed if they still didn't fit.

I summoned up all my courage and gathered up all my tightest jeans. I remember the jolt of glee I felt as I tried on a pair that never fit...the dreaded "red jeans". I had bought them a couple of years before and could only stuff myself into them one day back in Florida when I had been going to the gym 2 hours a day.

They were too tight even back then for me to wear in front of people. But this day, they slid up, buttoned and were even baggy on me! Oh My God!! I literally jumped up and down like a cheerleader! These were labeled size 12, but I always thought they had to be more like a 10.

Feeling so encouraged that all of my size 12 jeans were so loose; I decided to take the ultimate challenge. I went to my mother's room and asked if she had any size 10 jeans. She had always been smaller than me (and was vocally proud of the fact) so I knew she must have a pair.

She grudgingly handed me a pair of size 10 Liz Claiborne's that she hadn't been able to fit into for a long time (so she was doubly irritated).

I was nervous, but I forced myself to do it…I stepped in, pulled up, buttoned and zipped! Voile! It was as easy as could be! No tugging, squashing, laying down on the bed, doing lunges to stretch them out…no struggle at all! This was the ultimate day of my life! My mother's jeans! Oh Joy!

By the time of my 2-month follow up appointment, I was down to a glorious size 8 and had lost over 25 lbs.!   I had undergone ultrasound-assisted liposuction, which allows for very large volumes of fat to be removed at once. I will be forever grateful!

 To think that I got liposuction of my upper arms, back, waist, hips, butt, inner/outer/fronts and backs of my thighs…shrunk down from a size 14 to an 8 in just 2 months , all for only $1,500.00 total!! Pinch me…I've got to be dreaming!!!

 I am so happy with my new shape. He did such a great job…even sculpting a new butt for me! Now I have a nice, stylishly round hinee instead of the big flat 27" TV screen of a butt that I used to sit on!

The New Me!

Nearly 5 years later and I finally feel like the woman I was meant to be! I have gone from being a size 18 to being a size 2! I'm healthier, more energetic and self-confident. It's like my life is just starting fresh!

Words cannot express how good it feels to finally have won my life-long battle with fat. I threw out all of my dumpy-frumpy fat old lady clothes and replaced them with spunky new low-rise jeans and tight tank tops! I never, ever thought it was humanly possible for my body to wear a size 2!

I do not get teased about my weight anymore. In fact, my husband gave me the best compliment when he picked me up like a lady (instead of like a sack of potatoes like he used to) and said, "Look Sweetie! Now I can carry you femininily! Nobody could ever call you fat now!" (Yeah, he really said "fem-in-in-ily"…it was so cute ☺)

Wow…what a relief! To know that chapter of my life is over and I will never have to worry about gaining weight or feel guilty about every little morsel of food I put in my mouth! Yippee! It's like a dream come true for me.

I have a smoother, more pleasing and firmer shape. I can wear shorts or a bathing suit at the beach without feeling like some endangered species that has washed ashore, bloated and waterlogged. All and all, I am a much happier, more confident woman. I feel like I can take on the world…have, do or be whatever I choose! I feel free. Does that make me vain? No, it makes me normal. It makes me able to focus on my talents and gifts rather than my flaws. I don't feel like I have to hide to avoid being picked on. This is a milestone in my life. Sorry if it sounds like I'm bragging, but I'm so excited I want to shout it from the heavens!

It has been a long, sometimes painful, but totally rewarding journey. I have a new respect for my body, my life and my health. Exercise, once the horrid torture I inflicted upon myself, is now a joyful celebration of movement. No longer do I "hover" when my husband pulls me down to sit on his lap. I feel younger, stronger, more confident and capable in all areas of my life.

Recently, I mustered up the courage to wear a 2-piece swimsuit for the first time in my *ever*! And I felt beautiful! It made me remember when I was 10 years old and went to the ocean for the first time in Atlantic City, NJ. I was so self-conscious and embarrassed of being fat that I wore jeans. I actually wore *jeans* to the beach! That pretty much sums up the first 30 years of my life. Thanks to the excellent plastic surgery that I've been so lucky to receive, I'm not only sunning myself in a bikini in my Caribbean paradise, but I've even learned to swim, snorkel and scuba dive at the ripe old age of 35. Sure, I could have done those things when I was fat, but why open myself to the criticism and humiliation that I undoubtedly would have fallen victim to? I got enough of that when I was fully dressed!

My hope is that this book will help many, many people who have been cruelly teased about their big nose, flat chest, big gut, balding head, or thunder thighs and don't have $20,000.00 or $30,000.00 to spend on cosmetic surgery. Nor do you have to spend the last 20-30 years of your life looking elderly and infirm. I feel its time that we as a society stop treating cosmetic surgery as a shameful secret and embrace it as a modern means of physical maintenance. I predict that in the near future, the majority of people in our Western society will spend their 2-week vacations rejuvenating their bodies, minds and spirits, rather than wasting time and money standing in line to ride a rollercoaster then hitting the all-you-can-eat buffet.

I know that many people will tell you that you should accept yourself as God made you, ignore the vicious comments and injurious insults, and be "happy with who you are". It is true that we are all beautiful on the inside. It is also true that a beautiful spirit may wither with too many years of abuse.

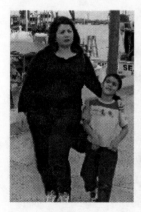 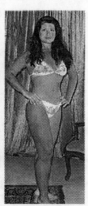

Unhappily Before   And Happily Ever After!

Who Are They to Judge, Anyway?

People who tell you that it is wrong to want to get cosmetic surgery either want to do it themselves and are too afraid, or want you to stay miserable for whatever personal reason they may have to keep you from feeling good about yourself.

Or perhaps they are lucky enough to be without any physical flaws, and have never had to endure the kind of bad treatment that many of us have. People like that could never understand why we want cosmetic surgery.

We live in a society where the eyes of every human being are fed images of beautiful, thin, gorgeous people every day for hours at a time. Unrealistic? Yes, of course. Can I change the media? Not a chance…but I do not have to allow myself to be on the outside looking in. In this glorious age, we possess the technology is to make us look better than nature has allowed.

And of course I don't mean to imply that looks are the most important thing in life. But the truth of our society remains. The beautiful people get all the breaks. And from what I've seen, chunky supermodels are still not coming into fashion, bald men are still not getting elected president, and elderly people are still not getting hired. I am not saying that I agree with the way things are, I am just saying…

If You Can't Beat Them, Join Them!

Cosmetic surgery is a trend that is showing no signs of slowing. The days of criticizing those of us who have had plastic surgery are soon to be gone for good.

I was once one of those who thought that plastic surgery was superficial and wasteful. It was how I was raised. I was also raised to think that a pint of ice cream was a single serving and that in America the president was elected by the people. You live, you learn.

The truth is, if you go around looking frumpy and dumpy you will feel frumpy-dumpy. You will probably lack confidence to get the things that you want in life. You will probably attract frumpy-dumpy people who don't light your fire. You will probably allow yourself to be treated badly, because frumpy-dumpy people get treated badly…it's just the way life is. You will probably settle for less than you deserve because when you look in the mirror you see a person who doesn't deserve the best.

Harsh words? Maybe, but the truth hurts sometimes. Now, I'm not saying that plastic surgery is the only way to look your best. I'm not even saying it's the best way! But it is a quick, effective way, usually with long-lasting results. It takes very little effort on your part, other than making the money to pay for it and having the guts to go through with it.

I don't mean to imply that you should undergo multiple procedures until you look like a Barbie doll. I don't want to live in a world where everybody looks the same, and I'm sure you feel that way, too. I'm sure you also don't want to live in a world where everybody looks like crap. Our society has a certain standard of beauty. We pretty much all respond to it the same way.

You may be thinking, 'But wait, JoAnn! What if EVERYBODY looks great? Then how will we be able to feel better than anybody else?' Geeze, would that be so bad? Maybe then we really could focus on our talents and gifts and individuality. Finally we would be able to get past the 'superficial', and love and admire each other for our inner unique qualities. It may be the long way around it, but perhaps we would finally stop being so mean to each other.

Think about it. What if everyone felt good about himself or herself? Don't you think there would be a whole lot less stress, anger, animosity and violence in the world? Am I going too far with this train of thought?

Sure, it takes a lot more to make you feel good about yourself than just knowing that you look your best. But let me tell you from experience, finally feeling good about your appearance after years of feeling ugly sure gets you a lot closer to Inner Peace.

Self-acceptance is more important than beauty, yet we all need to feel good about our physical presence. The physical, emotional and spiritual are all aspects of the one self that we have to nurture.

People form instant opinions just from the visual image that you present to them. It's human nature.

I wish people noticed my beautiful spirit when I walk in a room. Unfortunately, that's the very last thing anybody makes any time to look at. And if what they *are* noticing is not intriguing enough to spend any further time on…I'm out of luck.

Enough of my philosophizing about the importance of the physical; I would just like to encourage anyone who is considering cosmetic surgery to do your homework, check out the doctors you are considering, get your own physical health in peak condition, examine your own motivations, keep your expectations reasonable, and don't let fear block you from remedying your situation.

If you are reading this, there is no doubt that you are considering plastic surgery, for whatever reason.

I know all the fears you have from all the horror stories you have heard. Unfortunately because of the personal nature of plastic cosmetic surgery, people with horror stories are more vocal and eager to share their cosmetic surgery experiences than those of us who have had good plastic surgery and are happy with the results.

We happy cosmetic surgery patients want everyone to think that we "lost weight through willpower and determination", or just look younger because we changed our diet and exercise more, or our hair miraculously grew back on its own once we quit smoking or started to get more sleep!

The most successful plastic surgery is the surgery that makes you look better, but in an inconspicuous way.

Most cosmetic surgery veterans keep their successful surgeries as closely guarded secrets. It's fun to keep them guessing. Did she or didn't she? Isn't that selfish? Yes! I think so!

And I don't think that having cosmetic surgery is anything to be ashamed or embarrassed of, either. That is why I am willing to bare my soul and tell you the nitty gritty, where the best surgeons are, how to get good surgery you can afford and stop being left out of looking and feeling your best.

Why Should You Get Plastic Surgery?
You shouldn't! At least that is what many of your friends and relatives will tell you. In America, there is still a common underlying "stigma" about having plastic surgery…like if you choose to improve your appearance through surgery you are somehow vain and superficial. Yet, of all countries in the world, there is a constant worship of physical perfection in the USA.

It's a Catch-22 for sure.

I've heard it all a million times... "You should be happy the way you are...there are lots of people out there worse off than *you*!" -or- "You have to accept yourself the way God made you."

But let's get real...you never see even a slightly overweight person on TV or movies unless they are the butt of some joke (Teenage 'Monica' on "Friends"). Any girl that doesn't have ample knockers is picked on for being "flat" ('Grace' on "Will and Grace"). Then there's 'Ray' who is constantly picked on about his big nose on "Everybody Loves Raymond".

If you chat anonymously with someone new on the Internet, you inevitably get the $100,000 question... "So, R U Fat?" Even though the majority of Americans are severely overweight, this type of discrimination and degradation still prevails. It's so sad and destructive.

Yes, it would be wonderful if we could all just be happy with what we look like and content in the beauty of our souls. But the reality is our society does not allow it! That is the hard, cold truth. It's not about right or wrong, or what should or shouldn't be. It just is what it is and as each month passes it seems to get worse.

Statistics say that about 62% of Americans are now considered obese. That means that the majority of Americans are now overweight. Wouldn't you think that if the majority of people were a certain way that it would be considered "normal"? I can't figure it out, but I'm glad I don't have to dwell on it like I used to. Now I'm considered "normal", i.e. no longer overweight. But my heart still aches for those who are suffering like I did for all those years.

Competition is fierce...to get a job, to keep a job...to get a spouse, to keep a spouse...even just to get somebody to help you find a book in the library! Young, thin, good-looking people get all the attention. "Hey! That's not fair!" you say. I know, my friend... I feel your pain. But as your momma probably told you, life's not fair.

We are moving into an era where cosmetic surgery will soon be considered merely another chore in the average person's personal hygiene and physical maintenance routine. The stigma of plastic surgery is fading fast. It's become common knowledge that the lovely Demi Moore has spent over $330,000.00 on plastic surgery procedures to look perfect...some of it having been performed "overseas", although she hasn't disclosed where. However, she's living it up with her hot young stud, Ashton Kutcher, and obviously has no regrets.

Considering that we live the majority of our years as "old" (i.e. over 35), it is only natural that we should want to look good, if not great, for the majority of our lives. Stress, pollution, poor dietary and sleep habits plague our modern society and cause obvious physical ageing at ever-younger stages of life. Just as cosmetics and perfumes were once the vanities of the rich and uppity, then made affordable and acceptable to even the lowliest of serfs and peasants, so will be the course of acceptance for cosmetic surgery. Join me, won't you, in becoming the best looking peasants around? Just a little joke there, but you get my drift.

Plastic surgery is taking over the airwaves…It's not uncommon to see TV programs documenting the surgical procedures of the average man or woman, almost always ending with the unholy price tag of $15,000.00 or more. In fact, I saw a show the other day where a woman paid $40,000.00 just for a facelift and breast lift! But you don't have to pay these outrageous TV prices. Follow the advice in the pages that follow and you will save thousands, I promise!

There are lots of creative ways to finance your trip so you don't have to take any money out of your 401K or beg your parents for an advance on your inheritance. See my chapter, **"How to Make Sure Your Cosmetic Surgery is Painless…To Your Pocketbook!"** for some great ideas to create the cash you need to pay for your surgery.

At What Age is it Safe to Start Getting Lipo?

I recently asked my doctor what is the youngest age a patient can be for him to feel comfortable with performing liposuction. He told me it's perfectly safe and acceptable to perform liposuction on patients 15 years old and up.

My heart just sank when I heard those words. You see, when I was 15 I was a size 16. If I had known then what I know now, I would have been able to have my liposuction while I was still in High School! What a different life I would have had. It causes me such heartache to think of how I suffered and struggled trying to lose weight, hating my body and myself and feeling totally unlovable throughout my youth.

Well, it wasn't in the cards for me and perhaps that struggle has led me to my destiny. After all, had I not suffered for as long as I did I'm sure I would lack a lot of the compassion that I've developed toward my fellow plastic surgery seekers.

But if you have a child who is 15 or older and is struggling with a weight problem, please consider this option for him or her. You may save them years and years of emotional trauma and abuse by their social peers. I lived it, and I know the kind of silent pain that young, overweight people have to endure.

It is next to impossible for a young person to grow up with a healthy self-concept and live out their true potential when they are overweight. They are picked on and degraded on a regular basis by their classmates and even relatives, and they often have thoughts of suicide. I know I did.

I turned to alcohol and marijuana for a while as a means of escaping my inferiority complex, and I know a lot of other young people make the same mistake. The saddest thing about this avenue of escapism is that it leads to even more weight gain and depression.

I know that my stance on this issue of plastic surgery for teenagers may seem radical to you, and I have given it a lot of thought myself. But teenagers are getting meaner and meaner as the years go on, and being tormented at school on a regular basis is much more damaging to the human psyche than most parents are willing to admit. They opt for words of reassurance, ("its just baby fat. You'll grow out of it" or "Just go on a diet"). Words don't help, believe me. In fact, in most cases they just make the kid feel even worse.

Now, I'm not saying that I think you should force your 15-year-old to undergo surgery to remove 5 lbs. of belly fat. We should only opt for liposuction after all else has failed. Healthy diet and exercise work for some people, but have no effect on others.

But if you can see that your son or daughter has a chronic weight problem that is holding them back from blossoming into a healthy, well-adjusted adult I certainly think you should consider helping them get liposuction if he or she wants it.

Instead of shelling out a few thousand dollars on a crappy used car when she gets her driver's license, spend it on a good liposuction session and she won't mind walking to school or taking the bus.

Since I had the surgery I needed, I am now so much happier with my life! I want to help as many people as I can to feel great about themselves, too.

No one knows for sure how many tears are shed and talents are wasted over the superficial yet profound insecurities most of us suffer behind weight problems or other physical traits that others find unbecoming. I believe the plastic surgery revolution is in fact part of our human evolution. We are evolving into a charmed species…with the ability to improve ourselves physically, which will eventually lead to improving ourselves in every area of life.

After all, just think of all of the psychic, emotional and spiritual energy we waste over physical insecurity and unhappiness. When you feel great about yourself in every aspect of your life, there is no limit on what you can achieve.

You will no longer feel like you have to stay in an unhappy relationship for fear no one else will want you. You will start to look for the people and opportunities that you deserve, instead of those that are handed to you.

Going back to college will not be a horrifying idea once you get that facelift and look 10 or 15 years younger.

Taking your kids out for a walk will be more fun when you don't have to be concerned with getting a rash from your thighs rubbing together.

Think of this…when Oprah Winfrey was at her fattest, she admitted that she actually hoped that she DIDN'T win the Emmy Award she was nominated for that year because her butt was so big she didn't want to get up on stage in front of the world to show it off! Now that is sad. Don't let that be you! You must be ready to savor the moment when success comes your way!

It's not just beauty for beauty's sake, it is liberation from ugliness and that's got to be good!

So...How Cheap is Cheap?

In my research for this book, I interviewed several prominent Dominican plastic surgeons. When I brought up the issue of pricing, the reply was the same in each case. None of them were willing to give me a price per procedure. Their reason for this was that there is no "set price" for any procedure, as each case is reviewed on an individual basis.

A contributing factor to the unwillingness of the surgeons to give me "rough estimates" of what an individual procedure usually costs is that more often than not several procedures are performed at once, and the entire surgery is priced as one. They don't just add prices for each individual surgery together, but it is more a matter of the time and effort that goes into the procedure as a whole. And that means an excellent deal for you!

For example, when I had my tummy tuck my doctor told me that he felt that it was safe and prudent to do liposuction on my thighs and hips as well. The total price for everything was US$2,400.00. After some negotiation, the price went down to $1,800.00.

Although I went into some detail regarding negotiation in my first edition of this book, I no longer advise this. Times have changed, and this is really frowned upon these days. Haggling is a tricking business, and if you don't know how or when to do it properly it can be very offensive.

If you go to the Dominican Republic for surgery and choose a board certified surgeon, you will be getting an unbelievably low price for surgery performed by a highly skilled professional so I don't recommend getting petty over nickels and dimes, or even hundreds of dollars. When you are saving thousands, bickering over a couple of hundred is silly.

In my research on the Internet I found an average price for a tummy tuck in America is about $5,300.00 for the doctor's fee alone. The average liposuction cost is about $1,800.00 per area…that means if they perform liposuction on the outer thigh + the inner thigh + the hips it really means:

$1,800.00 x 3 = $5,400.00!

Add that to the tummy tuck and the total for everything that I had done would have cost around **$10,700.00** in the US.

That's not all I would have paid, however. The prices I have quoted above are the doctor's fees only! Normally the US patient will also be responsible for the cost of:

All operating room supplies = an extra fee ranging typically $500.00 to 1,500.00

Anesthesiologist = an extra fee ranging typically $500.00 to 1,500.00

Physical exam & blood work including HIV, liver function, hepatitis studies, thyroid tests, complete blood count—about 50 tests total, including electrocardiogram = $500.00

Follow-up visits x 3 = $150.00 to 250.00

In essence, if you have your surgery performed in the US you can pretty much count on it costing you at least $2,500.00 more than the price of the surgeon's fee (which is usually the price you will be originally quoted).

Of course, you will find doctors who will perform the surgery cheaper, some who will quote you with all costs included and still others who will quote you a much higher rate and attribute it to their "experience".
So...had I had my tummy tuck and liposuction in the US it would have cost:

10,700.00 in surgeon's fees
+ 2,500.00 additional fees/services
$13,200.00

But wait! I haven't included my 2-day hospital stay, which is about another $2,500.00 minimum.
$13,200.00
+ 2,500.00
$15,700.00

Wow! That is a far cry from the $2,400.00 price I found in the DR! As I mentioned earlier in this book, when you have surgery in the Dominican Republic (in all cases that I have ever heard about) the price your surgeon will give you is all-inclusive! You will not incur any other bills from hospitals, anesthesiologists, labs or any other ancillary services.

As another example, a reader asked me to get her a quote from my surgeon for a mini-facelift including upper and lower eyelids as well as autologous chin implant. She had an online consultation with a plastic surgeon in New Jersey who quoted her a price of $12,500.00. The price my surgeon offered to do the same work for was…$2,400.00! She had my surgeon perform the surgery, got AWESOME results (I saw her before and after, so I know) and she **saved over $10,000.00** on her surgery!

I recently spoke with her, and she told me that she was thrilled with the results of her Dominican facelift, but she was embarrassed to admit that she had just gotten liposuction on her stomach in the United States that she paid $5,000.00 for and was very unhappy with her results. She experienced a lot of pain and didn't get the results that she had expected. She now wishes that she had come back to the Dominican Republic for her liposuction since she would have been able to get liposuction in multiple areas and still would have saved a couple of thousand dollars!

Another reader asked me to get her a quote for breast enlargement, neck lift and rhinoplasty (nose job). All of these surgeries together performed in the United States would have cost her a minimum of $16,000.00 (and that's absolute minimum). The quote I got for her was only $4,800.00!

Even if you were to add another $4,000.00 for an all-inclusive luxury vacation including gourmet meals (lobster and shrimp every day if you want), 24-hour personal assistant, manicures, pedicures, massage, and private ground transportation service you would still save over $7,000.00!!

Keep in mind, my surgery was performed by one of the best plastic surgeons in the country, and the price was still that low. Take into consideration that all of the Dominican plastic surgeons that I am including in this book are real plastic surgeons, not dermatologists, dentists or other doctors presenting themselves as cosmetic surgeons, as is common in the United States.

In case you weren't aware, even in America with very minimal training any kind of doctor can present himself as a "cosmetic surgeon", but that does not make him a "plastic surgeon". Cosmetic surgeons can only perform certain procedures and do not have the intense training and experience in plastic and reconstructive surgery that true accredited plastic surgeons have.

DOMINICAN PLASTIC SURGERY PRICES

Dr. Roberto Guerrero was kind enough to provide me with a list of prices for several of his most requested surgeries. Please keep in mind that these are the "ballpark figures", i.e. average estimated costs.

Each individual patient is different and requires treatment as such, so if you need more than the average amount of surgery your final price will of course be somewhat higher. However, these figures will give you a fairly good idea of what to expect.

Also, often when a patient is having more than one procedure at one time, the patient will be quoted a combined price that is lower than simply adding the base prices of each procedure together. Therefore, if you plan to have several procedures performed at once, you stand to save a TON of money...like I did!

PLASTIC SURGERY COSTS – US vs. DR	Average US Surgeon Fees Only (Additional Operating Costs are Added Separately)	Dominican Republic All-Inclusive Surgery Cost
LIPOSUCTION	$7224.00 (one area only)	$3000.00 MULTIPLE AREAS!
ABDOMINOPLASTY (tummy tuck)	$8250.00	$2500.00
FACELIFT	$8500.00	$4000.00
BUTTOCK LIFT	$10,000.00	$2000.00
BREAST ENLARGE	$8750.00	$3000.00
BREAST REDUCTION	$7857.00	$2200.00
GYNECOMASTIA (male breast reduction)	$6939.00	$2000.00
RHINOPLASTY (Nose)	$7188.00	$2200.00
CHIN AUGMENTATION	$5693.00	$2000.00

OTOPLASTY (Ears)	$6535.00	$2000.00
BRACHIOPLASTY (Upper Arm Lift)	$6809.00	$2000.00
THIGHPLASTY (Thigh lift)	$7283.00	$2500.00

How Can I Get Quality Cosmetic Surgery So Cheap?

If there's one thing that makes me absolutely cringe, it's when I read articles about medical tourism and overseas plastic surgery that refer to the prices as "cut-rate". Nothing could be further from the truth! This implies that the prices are purposely set low for Americans to lure them to other countries or because the quality is not up to par with American standards. What a crock!

It's all a matter of simple economics. You see, your American dollar is worth between 30-35 Dominican Pesos! (The exchange rate changes daily). That means that your money goes a lot further here! Plus, it is much less expensive overall to live here, so doctors and hospitals don't have to charge the exorbitant prices that their American counterparts do.

Another important contributing factor is the fact that Dominican Society is not as litigious (eager to sue) as American Society. Because there is not the need for exorbitant malpractice insurance coverage, the surgeons do not have to charge such ridiculously high prices as in the States and most of UK and Europe. The savings, as they say, are passed on to you!

The Dominican doctors listed in this book are board certified by the Dominican Society of Plastic and Reconstructive Surgeons (Sociedad Dominicana de Cirugía Plastica Y Reconstructiva, Inc.) and are held to extremely high standards, just like certified plastic surgeons in the United

States and Europe. Sanitation codes and practices are the same (if not better) than in the States.

See my chapter **"How to Choose A Plastic Surgeon in the Dominican Republic"** for details. They keep up on all the latest medical and surgical advances and technology. In fact, because Dominican society is much more open to innovations used in Europe and South America, often times state of the art techniques, products and medications are being utilized here that are not available in the U.S.

When I say that cosmetic surgery in the Dominican Republic, is all-inclusive... it means that you pay one time for everything including: preoperative visit and surgical consultation, your blood work, the surgery itself, the nursing staff, the hospital stay, pain medication, compression garments, the anesthesiologists, food, even the follow up doctor's visits!

You will not get bill after bill in the mail for months following your surgery (like in the US).

How to Make Sure Your Cosmetic Surgery is Painless...To Your Pocketbook

Since I've already explained that it's really cheap to get good quality cosmetic plastic surgery in the Dominican Republic, I would like to help you finance your surgery without spending any of your savings or creating any more debt on your credit cards.

By now, I am sure that you have heard of eBay, the online auction web site. You probably have either bought or sold something there already. If not, I have to tell you that it is easy and extremely profitable. My husband and I have been members of eBay since 1998, and we have made literally thousands of dollars by selling things on eBay!

What did we sell? Everything and anything! We have even bought things on eBay and resold them on eBay for a profit! It sounds incredible, but I can't tell you how many times we would be tight on cash...not even being able to pay the month's bills...and we would put an ad on eBay to sell something we had lying around the house or garage that we no longer used and BINGO! We made enough money to pay the bills!

Believe me, it takes a lot of guilt out of the process when you don't have to rack up more debt on the family credit cards or spend money that you had earmarked for your retirement or the kids' education!

One example of how my husband and I made extra money for quite a while on eBay. I was a medical transcriptionist for 7 years. I knew that in many areas of the country, a good used transcription machine at a good price was hard to find.

I was spotting some really good, cheap ones on eBay every once in a while that were advertised badly, usually being sold by people who didn't even know what they were for or how much they were worth! I would buy them for $5.00 to $10.00 dollars each and resell them on eBay or on medical transcription web site classified ads for $80.00 to $100.00 each! That's a great profit with very little work involved.

And after that, it was so funny, because it seemed like these things were showing up everywhere we went! We would go to computer shows and flea markets, and people would be giving them away! They'd say, "I don't even know what the heck it's for…Take it! Give me a buck or two, that's all!" Wow, what a trip!

It was just a matter of having some "inside information" to recognize value where others didn't! And I helped a lot of people in the process who did not want to pay $200.00 or $300.00 on a new machine. It was a win-win situation all around and I got a lot of nice thank you notes as a result!

We have also bought loose diamonds, got official appraisals, had them set in nice ring or earring settings and resold them on eBay for 200-300% profits! No kidding! It paid for all of our Christmas shopping a couple of years ago!

I tell this to you friend to friend…the potential to make money on eBay is only limited by your own willingness to spend a little time (very little) and just doing it! It can be so much fun to watch the price of your item going up and up! Now that I think about it, I should have something on eBay right now. Sometimes I forget how much fun it is!

I encourage you to use eBay to create some money "out of the blue" for yourself. Going to yard sales and buying TV's for $25.00 and reselling them on eBay for $75.00 or $100.00. Flea market finds that the seller will practically give away can become instant cash in your pocket if you know how to use eBay and how to create a good ad!

The money for your surgery can pile up fast. Selling on eBay is inexpensive, and now that it is so amazingly successful it is the cheapest form of advertising the world has ever known! You may find yourself an entirely new business in the process!

Another tool I have used to generate positive cash flow in a short amount of time was Stuart Lichtman's **"How to Get Lots of Money for Anything…FAST!"** The results I achieved using Mr. Lichtman's Cybernetic Transposition techniques were nothing short of AMAZING! It seemed like a lot of money to spend at the time, but I knew it was an investment that would pay for itself…and I was right!

Using these techniques, I created a "metastory"…a situation that I wanted to happen to bring me something (money and publicity) that I needed. Not a week later, I was contacted out of the blue by a freelance writer from England who wanted to do a story on me and my book to be published in the UK's **"Woman"** magazine!

Not only would I get fabulous publicity for my book, but also they were going to pay me the equivalent of $500.00 for my interview! I couldn't believe it! Just days before, I sat and wrote my metastory that I would write an article and get it published in newspapers and magazines and subsequently get tons of traffic and sales from my web site. Not only did I get what I wanted, but also I didn't even have to write the article myself!

I highly recommend that you try the methods in **"How to Get Lots of Money for Anything…FAST!"** It is amazing. And it comes with lots of bonuses and streaming audio seminar segments that aren't even advertised! I've learned so much about how your subconscious mind can actually prevent you from getting the things you want, and how to "rework" a situation so that both your conscious and subconscious minds are driven to get you what you want. This is powerful stuff.

How do I choose a Plastic Surgeon in the Dominican Republic?

Just like in America, you should always choose a doctor who is "Board Certified". Similar to the United States' American Medical Association (AMA), the Dominican Republic holds it's medical doctors to the highest standard through various medical associations, including the Dominican Medical Association (Asociación Médica Dominicana), the Ibero-Latina American Federation (Federación Ibero Latinoamericana), and specific to the field of Plastic Surgery is the **Dominican Society of Plastic and Reconstructive Surgeons** (Sociedad Dominicana de Cirugía Plástica Y Reconstructiva).

Again, as in the United States, in order to become a board certified plastic surgeon, a medical doctor (having earned a university degree in medicine and earned title of practicing doctor of medicine) must complete two years of residency in general surgery, followed by an additional three years residency in plastic surgery.

In addition, to become a member of the Dominican Society of Plastic and Reconstructive Surgeons, the surgeon must adhere to strict guidelines as set by the Society, including constant continuing educational courses and conferences. He or she must also conduct their practice in the highest ethical fashion to continue membership.

The purpose of the Dominican Society of Plastic and Reconstructive Surgeons is to guarantee the patient that if he/she chooses to undergo surgery by a surgeon who is a member of the Society, he/she will receive the highest quality of care and surgical skill.

To emphasize, you should always choose a plastic surgeon who is a member of the Dominican Society of Plastic and Reconstructive Surgeons as this is your only means to know for sure that he or she is well-trained and held to the highest standards.

The more plastic surgery societies that the doctor is a member of, the better. Being a member of many of these organizations proves that the doctor is concerned and dedicated to staying active in his field and keeping his own standards and practices as high as possible.

How do I choose amongst the members of the Dominican Society of Plastic and Reconstructive Surgeons?

Important criteria to take into consideration when choosing your surgeon include the following:

If you don't speak Spanish (well or at all), make sure you choose a surgeon who speaks English.

Do you have any friends or associates who can recommend a surgeon to you from personal experience with that doctor? If not, is the surgeon that you are considering able to provide you with phone numbers of any of his previous patients or before and after pictures?

Do you like his/her general attitude? Does he/she make you feel comfortable and confident in your choice?

Is this surgeon willing to take the time to explain to you the details of the procedure and give you a good understanding of the risks involved?

Does the surgeon encourage you to ask questions?

Does he/she seem realistic and conscientious in the results offered?

Does the surgeon put your health and welfare in highest priority?

Does the surgeon have an Internet email address through which you can communicate with him and send him pictures of yourself, so he can better plan your surgery and offer surgical advice?

Does the surgeon publish his Curriculum Vitae on the Internet or in a brochure so you can review his credentials and education?

Communicating With Your Dominican Republic Plastic Surgeon

I do not speak Spanish fluently, although at this point I can understand a lot of what is being said. At the time that I had my surgery, I knew a lot less Spanish and had a tendency to just smile a lot and totally block out what was being said around me! Luckily, however, many of the plastic surgeons in the Dominican Republic do speak and understand English fairly well and some are very fluent in English, so that was not the big issue that I thought it would be.

For some people though, it would be distressing to not be able to communicate perfectly with the secretaries, nurses and other medical staff. If you are one of those people, you would be best off to find a friend who speaks both languages well and keep them close at hand!

You may think that this is not an option for you, but it is not as difficult as you may think. I have total confidence that via the Internet forums and chat rooms you could make such a friend.

You could meet a "Surgery Buddy" through my forum at **http://www.cheap-plastic-surgery.com/InvisionBoard.html** or on one of the many other Internet plastic or cosmetic surgery forums. I highly suggest making friends with other like-minded people for emotional support before, during and after your cosmetic surgery procedure.

I have benefited highly from my alliances with my new Internet friends who shared my concerns, fears and joys. There's just no substitute! Surrounding yourself only with people who just don't understand what you are going through or do not support your decision can be devastating.

The other option you have for overcoming the language barrier you may encounter by having your surgery in the Dominican Republic is to learn Spanish. I suggest this to everyone anyway considering the fact that more and more of the American population is Spanish-speaking.

Speaking the Spanish language fluently will help you in your work almost undoubtedly in one way or another, could get you a better job than the one you have and will open up the doors of love or friendship with some of the nicest people in the world!

Learning to communicate in Spanish also will make you more confident when traveling to countries where Spanish is the national language. The good thing about Spanish is that it uses almost all of the same letters as English and so many of the words are so similar to English words of the same meaning, it's not nearly as difficult as learning most languages of the world. Some great low-cost or free tutorials are available on the Internet.

At the end of this book, I have included a list of Spanish phrases that you should know if you have surgery in a Spanish-speaking country. These phrases are invaluable and not difficult to remember. And learning them will take a lot of stress out of the experience. I have also included links to my favorite online Spanish tutorials.

What are the risks involved with Plastic Surgery?

Although most people consider plastic surgery to be less risky than most other types of surgery, there are still many risks. In fact, Plastic Surgery shares all of the same inherent risks as any general surgery procedure along with the risk of physical disability in the form of numbness, tingling and loss of sensation and/or muscle paralysis, bleeding, infection, scarring, complications from anesthesia (including death), etc.

In short, plastic surgery is nothing to be taken lightly. It is surgery, and you had best be sure that the risks do not outweigh the potential benefits.

Because of the nature of cosmetic surgery and the motivation behind wanting to undergo such procedures, the prospective patient should seek to balance her own emotional state and examine her psychological needs and expectations.

Cosmetic surgery is a very intimate and personal experience. Many people expect that changing the physical will cure the emotional pain they may suffer. This is not always the outcome of having plastic surgery. In fact, the patient could experience deep emotional pain following even the most successful cosmetic procedure.

Bottom line…there is no "quick fix" to a traumatized mind. Please see the chapter **"Use Your (Recovery) Time Wisely"**, which offers ideas on healing and strengthening the emotional, psychological and spiritual self that you can benefit from both pre- and post-surgery.

That being said, there are many things that you can do to physically prepare yourself for surgery and help minimize risks.

Few people, especially Americans, take responsibility for their own health prior to seeing any type of doctor for any reason. There is a general attitude of "that's what doctors are for". In fact, most Americans don't see a doctor until they are ill. It should not be that way!

You owe it to yourself to learn how your body works, what it needs to run properly and how to protect your health from illness, fatigue and disease. YOU are smart enough to learn basic biology and preventative medicine.

Most doctors would like you to believe that only *they* have the capacity to understand what makes the human body tick and how to treat disease and fight infection.

The truth is that the average person is fully capable of comprehending the principals of good health and initiating simple good habits that promote health.

I want to encourage you to learn about how to keep your body in optimal health. If you are full of pathogens that are lying dormant, waiting until a time when you are weak enough for them to wreak havoc on your body, you are already at risk for complications during your surgery.

What are the Risks of Having My Surgery Performed in the Dominican Republic?

You will find articles on the web discouraging you from seeking surgery in countries other than the United States.

The reasons for the articles are clearly to protect the practices of American cosmetic and plastic surgeons. They are well aware that the lower prices available for cosmetic surgery in other countries of the world are a huge incentive for their potential patients to look elsewhere.

If you are in good physical and mental health prior to surgery and you go to a qualified plastic surgeon in any country with proper medical standards, and stay there long enough to get through your initial recovery time (at least 2 weeks), you should have no problem.

In fact, if you look on any cosmetic surgery message board you will find lots of examples of patients who had surgery by doctors in the US, were dissatisfied with the outcome and the doctor would not even take their phone calls afterward!

Just because you have your surgery done by an American doctor does not insure that your outcome will be good or that you will get adequate after-care. You take chances by having cosmetic surgery anywhere you go.

Most Dominican Republic plastic surgeons frequently travel to the United States and Europe to attend medical conferences and training programs, meet and consult with potential new patients and to check in on past patients.

And, the Dominican Republic is so close to America; on the off chance you should need to have any type of touch-up procedure it's not such a big deal.

In my experience of three separate surgery sessions performed by two different Dominican Republic Plastic Surgeons in two different clinics, I found standards and practices to be just as high or higher than those of the 4 hospitals that I worked at in the United States over a 7-year period when I worked as a medical transcriptionist.

Another one of my readers is a Registered Nurse in the United States and she had surgery performed at the same clinic and by the same doctor as I did, and she felt the same way. She was very happy with everything…and she didn't tell anyone ahead of time that she was an RN, so she received no special treatment based on her professional status.

I tell you all this because I want to reiterate that I am **NOT** recommending that you go to a grass hut where they hit you over the head with a mallet as a form of anesthesia and cut you open with a kitchen knife because it will save you thousands of dollars.

Please don't ask your surgeon if they sterilize their instruments or screen blood for transfusions. They will find it very offensive that you would assume that they would be so ignorant as to neglect these common medical standards!

These are **HIGHLY TRAINED MEDICAL PROFESSIONALS!** Don't insult them by implying that they don't know or care about common sterilization techniques and preventing disease. Just because they live and work in a small country does not mean that they are crude or retarded. And just because you read the newspaper and watch TV does not mean you know more than they do.

Like I wrote earlier, they all have thriving practices and they don't *need* you as a patient. You need them! If you take a haughty attitude you will make them not want to work with you. Try not to come off as an "Arrogant American".

If you do treat them with any less respect that you would treat an American surgeon, I will most likely start getting phone calls asking me to remove their names from my book.

It is best for you to be as easy to deal with and as respectful as possible. Now, I don't mean that you shouldn't ask questions and be aware of what is happening to you. Your health is my main concern.

However, I do hope that you inform yourself as much as possible on your own by reading all of the information you can about the procedure you are having done, and just don't make yourself a nuisance.

If you are spending a lot of time trying to find reasons why you *shouldn't* have surgery here or anywhere else for that matter, then don't do it!

You are not a good candidate for surgery if you are purposely trying to freak yourself out about it. Keep dieting or accept the fact that you are starting to look old. When I finally was able to get my plastic surgery, I was in the mindset of, "Anything will be better than where I'm at today. I just can't go on the rest of my life fighting this losing battle".

You have to have a certain amount of trust and a certain amount of desperation to undergo elective cosmetic surgery. That may not sound appealing to you, but it is the honest truth.

Your mind is very, very powerful. If you dwell on negative thoughts, you will create a negative experience for yourself no matter what. If you expect the worst, you will create the worst.

A positive attitude and proactive approach are the keys to success in every avenue of life, but especially when it comes to elective cosmetic surgery.

Overseas surgery is a great option for those who (like me) are at their wits end, want good plastic surgery performed by Board Certified Plastic Surgeons and don't have the money or credit to go to the doctor down the street!

It is also the ideal option for those who DO NOT want friends, family and business associates to know they are having plastic surgery. When you go to the Dominican Republic for plastic surgery, your anonymity is built-in to the process. You don't have to hide in your house for two or three weeks and hope nobody you know drops by to visit! You just return from your Caribbean vacation looking fabulous.

Please don't email the doctors 10 or 20 times asking common sense questions. These are busy professionals and time is money. Please keep your questions concise, appropriate and try to keep the number of emails as few as possible.

Save any hemming and hawing for lunch with your girlfriends. It is not part of the doctor's job to talk you into having surgery. He should be open and honest about details of the procedures and any risks involved, but ethically should not try to convince you if you are unsure of whether you want to have surgery or not.

If you approach him in this manner, they may just tell you that he won't be your doctor. And I really wouldn't blame them.

I am sorry to have to make this point so strongly, but I have gotten feedback from doctors who are telling me horror stories in this regard.

I am afraid that if it continues, they will start raising their prices just to compensate for the extra time they have to spend answering emails and phone calls.

Again, please keep your emails to sending photos and scheduling consultations, and do as much general research about plastic surgery as possible on your own.

I myself have been bombarded with questions regarding plastic surgery, which I try to cheerfully answer.

And at the same time I have been criticized for charging for my book! It is very strange why some people think that I should expend such tireless efforts for free. Who works for free? Everybody has to pay the bills. Please be respectful of that. Cheap does not mean free.

The doctors, clinics and hospitals here in DR operate under strict health codes and are very careful. The ladies who recommended the plastic surgeons I went to are extremely wealthy and could have had their plastic surgery anywhere they desired. They fly to New York just to do a little shopping! Yet they chose to have their surgery here. That was enough convincing for me.

HOW TO AVOID WOUND INFECTION

The issue of wound infection is one that has become quite controversial in recent months. The Health Commissioner of NYC put out a "Health Alert" in recent months because 9-11 women who had undergone plastic surgery in the Dominican Republic developed Mycobacterium Abscessus infections following their return to the United States.

The amount of slanted news stories and misinformation that flooded the media regarding these infections was horrendous. I kept track of the stories, and did extensive research regarding this type of infection and I can tell you that I honestly believe that the entire situation was blown out of proportion drastically for one reason…the plastic surgeons of New York City and the United States in general are getting very, very nervous. They know how many people are becoming aware of the affordable options now available to them by having their surgery performed in the Dominican Republic.

I have been very careful not to jump to these conclusions. I explored the CDC's (Center for Disease Control – US) own web site and found that the source of infection, Mycobacterium Abscesus, is NOT a rare strain of bacteria unique to the Dominican Republic, as the Health Commissioner and others in NYC erroneously stated. It is a common source of infection world-wide, and more importantly in the United States!

In fact, again according to the CDC's own web site, the bacteria found responsible for the infections in these 9 ladies (called Mycobacterium abscessus), "is found in water, soil and dust." The patients could have just as easily contracted the infections in their own homes. This "health alert" made by these local politicians are not only premature, but sorely lacking in concrete evidence. But it is easy to make damning statements with little or no basis in fact when the victims of such accusations (the Plastic Surgeons of the Dominican Republic) are in another country.

Of course, the recent death of well-known American author Olivia Goldsmith while undergoing plastic surgery in Manhattan has shed a glaring and unflattering light on the quality and safety (or lack thereof) of plastic surgery in the United States. Ms. Goldsmith was undergoing surgery at the Manhattan Eye, Ear and Throat Hospital, where she had cardiac arrest following induction of general anesthesia, which the hospital referred to as a "known complication". According to WNBC, "A second patient died at Manhattan Eye, Ear and Throat Hospital on Feb. 16 after she was erroneously given an anesthesia injection in her larynx, the medical examiner's office said. In May, the state health department fined the hospital $20,000 for breakdowns in patient care in anesthesia and plastic surgery."

In order to recede back into the shadows and hopefully counteract the impending mass exodus of plastic surgery patients from America to the Dominican Republic, a "movement" has been formed to attempt to blow-up a few untoward post-surgical infections into a "health alert". Had these infections occurred in New Jersey or Idaho (as they do each and every day), they certainly would not be the fodder for a "Health Alert".

I, for one, know first hand that there are excellent plastic surgeons and top-notch medical facilities in the Dominican Republic and I have absolutely no qualms about recommending it to other Americans who, like me, need and want quality plastic surgery and do not want to pay the outrageous prices in the United States. Instead of pointing the finger at other countries and creating panic and mistrust where none is warranted, the Healthcare System in the United States should make the effort to raise the bar and improve their own level of competency, safety and affordability. The old adage "You get what you pay for" most certainly does not apply where American plastic surgery is concerned. You can be sure that Ms. Goldsmith certainly did not get what she paid for.

The type of complications and infections that the "Health Alert" warned of, occur in thousands of patients in America each year. Convincing the public that they are safer by having their surgery in the United States as opposed to going to the Dominican Republic is irresponsible, misleading, and slanderous against many highly skilled and talented Dominican Republic plastic surgeons.

There is no evidence presented by this "Health Alert" to support the assumption that having surgery in the US is any safer than having it in the Dominican Republic. The truth is, according to the Center for Disease Control's own web site:

"(In the United States) Postoperative surgical site infections remain a major source of illness and a less frequent cause of death in the surgical patient). These infections number approximately 500,000 per year..."

Additionly, in recent years the Journal of the American Medical Association (JAMA 2000 Jul 26;284 (4):483-5.) published an article proclaiming that doctors and hospitals were the 3rd leading cause of death in America!

In fact, I discovered that there were 2 cases documented of the same infection resulting from soft tissue augmentation performed right in New York City back in 2003, as published in the National Library of Medicine (PMID: 12930343 [PubMed - indexed for MEDLINE]) , as well as: "14 confirmed and 11 suspected cases in New York City of M abscessus infection after illicit cosmetic procedures. As injectable cosmetic procedures are becoming increasingly popular, dermatologists should be aware of both the common and unusual complications. Furthermore, all physicians should be alerted to the current cluster of M abscessus infections after injections for cosmetic purposes by nonmedical practitioners in New York City."
PMID: 14988690 [PubMed - in process]

So, why was there no "health alert" made urging people not to have injectable cosmetic procedures in the United States? Or at the very least, not to get them in New York City? Another Mycobacterial outbreak occurred in Northern California in May of 2003, where over 100 patrons of a salon came down with the infection following pedicures (Arch

Dermatol. 2003 May;139(5):629-34.). Should all Americans have been put on "health alert" and warned not to get pedicures in the state of California? Well no, of course not…that would be silly, wouldn't it?

It is only obvious that the recent deluge of bad press regarding plastic surgery in the Dominican Republic is supporting a political agenda…the attempt to bring an end to the increasing numbers of US citizens who are leaving the country to get the high-quality plastic surgery that they want at a reasonable price that they can afford.

Let me tell you one important thing, we are all bombarded by millions of bacteria and viruses each day.

Our bodies are amazingly efficient at destroying most of these pathogens without our conscious minds even knowing we've been exposed to them.

When you undergo surgery, dental work, physical trauma and even mental stress/distress, your immune system (the body's germ fighting mechanism) is weakened. It is of utmost importance that you do all you can to strengthen your body and your immune system at all times, but especially prior to any surgery.

As I mentioned before in this text, any surgery you undergo puts you at risk of developing infection. Your doctor will undoubtedly prescribe a course of peri-surgical antibiotics to help kill off any pathogens that are already lurking in your body before your surgery, as well as those you may encounter during and after surgery.

Also, I have always been prescribed a course of Vitamin C following my surgery. Vitamin C is nature's immune booster and it is very effective. I highly suggest using it on a regular basis, but especially pre- and post surgery.

As mentioned earlier, cleansing your body (i.e. liver, kidney, bowel and parasite cleanses) will greatly improve your overall health and kill most or all of those pathogens that make you sick and cause infections.

Another item I have added to my arsenal of defense against pathogens is a Zapper. A zapper is a small electronic box with wristbands or other electrodes that you apply to your body and wear for an allotted amount of time (7 minutes on, 20 minutes off times 3 cycles).

The zapper runs on a simple 9-volt battery, and sends a current through your body that you usually do not feel (except maybe a little tingling). This current is mild enough not to have any negative effect on the body's own cells, yet it runs at a frequency that kills a multitude of germs, bacteria and even viruses.

I have used my zapper with amazing results many, many times. In fact, every time my son starts to get the sniffles or a cough, I have him zap for an hour and his symptoms disappear...without a drop of medicine!

A very nice elderly lady who lives down the street from me here in the Dominican Republic experienced one of the most astounding results I have personally seen from zapping. I was so impressed by her healing that I posted a full account on the Curezone web site. Below I have included my post.

Subject: The Zapper Works!
From: Jmrros |
Date: 1/21/2003 9:18:38 AM
I live in the Dominican Republic (recently moved from Florida).

I met a sweet lady of about 72 years of age who told me she had been suffering with pain and atrophy of her left thumb and wrist for 8 years.

Her hand was bent and crippled; she could no longer use it. In addition, she had a large open sore on the tip of her middle finger (same hand) that would not heal. She had the sore for over a year and a half! It was scary looking, to say the least.

She went to the United States to see a "specialist". This cost her a small fortune. He put her on antibiotics and told her that she had suffered some injury (she insists she did not), and that there was nothing else he could do for her. She was going to have to live with it. She took the antibiotics until the prescription ran out, but nothing changed.

I was quite intimidated when my husband told her I could help. I have studied Dr. Clark's books for about a year and am a true believer in her work, but I don't talk to many people about it because of the negative reaction that most people have to anything that contradicts the

Establishment.

I gave her my zapper and told her to zap for an hour a day and to soak her finger in an Epsom salt bath every day.

To my delight, her finger was completely healed in about 2 weeks!!! Her hand is now totally free of pain and she can use it fine. In fact, the areas of muscle wasting in the thenar eminence (muscles of the palm-thumb area) have built themselves back up! They were caved in and wasted.

She is so happy! She thinks I am a genius! The credit goes to Dr. Clark, though. That is for sure. I just feel so wonderful to have helped someone heal like that. I have had many other "minor miracles" with the use of the zapper in my family, but this one was so visible and profound, I had to share it!

END POST

At the end of this book, I have listed some sites where you can read more about zappers, buy zappers, and get free plans to build your own zapper if you are electronically inclined.

Yet another underestimated (and practically unheard of in the United States) electrical device that kills bacteria, viruses, germs, molds, mildew and even nasty odors is an ozonator. I literally have four of these things in my house and I love them all!

Ozonators create ozone…yes, *that ozone*; the layer with the hole in it. Ozone is actually 3 atoms of oxygen that temporarily stick together; thus the symbol for ozone, which is O3.

Ozone has been used for over 40 years in Germany and other parts of Europe to treat many afflictions, and is currently being used effectively in killing HIV. Although there are a few different methods of treatment using ozone, the easiest for home use is drinking ozonated water. The ozonator I use is a small portable system that is housed in a plastic tackle box. The unit has a hose and a bubbler (like on a tropical fish tank).

Ozone is extremely effective in killing pathogens. I have a super-powerful ozonator in my living room to clean the air, a small unit that is made for the refrigerator (awesome), and another unit in the bathroom that is made to sterilize the toothbrushes, razors and other personal care items.

At the end of the book you'll find lots of links to web sites that have more information about the amazing power of ozone, places where you can buy your own ozonators, as well as places where you can go to receive professional ozone therapy treatments.

Prior to your surgery, do an extremely thorough housecleaning, of your body and your home. When you return home from your surgery, it is important that your heavy cleaning is done.

You will not be up to doing it post-op…nor should you! The physical stress will not be good for your healing process, and the dust and critters you stir out of the corners can cause infection.

Germs collect in dust, dirt and kitchen grease. Give your refrigerator a thorough cleaning, too. Make sure there are no molds growing anywhere.

If you have household pets, try to keep them outside if you can. If you can't, try not to pet or cuddle with them for as long as you can stand it…at least until your wounds are completely healed and free of redness.

If you can't resist petting your pooch, please wash your hands with hot, soapy water immediately after. Don't let the cats or dogs sleep in your bedroom. Do not clean the cat litter box yourself. Have somebody else do it, preferably wearing disposable rubber gloves.

If you have a baby or young child at home, it is imperative that you have someone else change the diapers and clean up the ca-ca until your surgical wounds are completely healed, at least 6 weeks following your surgery. If this is not an option, then I strongly advise you to wait a couple of years to have your surgery until your children are more capable of wiping their own bottoms.

For even more hints and tips on how to keep your external and internal environment clean and healthy please refer to Dr. Hulda Clark's book, **"The Cure for All Diseases"**. Once you read this book, you will no longer go through life fearing disease and illness! The knowledge you will gain about the nature of illness will empower you!

I come from a town where cancer is a plague...in fact 11 of my family members have suffered from various forms and/or died horrible deaths from cancer including my father at age 48, both of my grandmothers, some cousins, aunts and uncles. I was terrified of it myself until I read Dr. Clark's books.

That is why I recommend so strongly that you spend at least 6 weeks (2 months is best) doing all you can to purify your internal environment prior to surgery...any type of surgery.

One of the first and most important steps is colon cleansing. It's an area that we're all grossed out about, and never want to even mention, but it is the gateway to good health. If the internal walls of your intestinal tract are coated in old fecal material, you've not only got a breeding ground for the nasties, you are also preventing all of the nutrients from your food from being absorbed into the blood stream! It's a double whammy.

Most people don't realize that our modern American diet turns to a thick, gummy paste inside our bodies and sticks to the walls of the intestines like rubber cement. We eat so few vegetables and fruits, natures "wall-scrubbers", that this goop just builds up and builds up until the intestines are barely functioning. Instead of the normal peristaltic reaction that pushes digested food through the instine quickly and efficiently, food is pushed through by the next food you put on top of it.

I don't think I need to go into that part of it any further. Let's now get on to how you can effectively cleanse your colon without having to suffer any humiliating enemas. Don't get me wrong, I'm sure enemas are the most effective way to do a thorough colon cleansing. However, it's not something I can bring myself to do. Too embarrassing and I'm too self-conscious for that. I can barely stand a pedicure because of the thought of another human scraping stuff out from under my toenails.

Here is the recipe for the absolute best way to cleanse your colon and make yourself feel better than you have in years! And the most fantastic part is that all these ingredients are cheap and easy to get, and you don't have to stick a hose up your butt!

INGREDIENTS:

Psyllium Husk Powder

Psyllium Husks, Whole

Bentonite Calcium Clay Powder

Diatomaceous earth

Dr. Hulda Clark's Black Walnut Hull Tincture

Ground fresh papaya seeds

Caprylic Acid capsules

Tumeric, Powder (a yellow spice)

Cayenne Pepper (the hottest BTU's you can find)

Freshly squeezed or extracted fruit juice (any kind)

Okay, fill a large glass half-way up with your juice. Add 2 big tablespoons of an even mixture of the Bentonite clay and Diatomaceous earth and mix rapidly. Now add 1/4 tsp. of the Cayenne and Turmeric. Add 1/2 tsp. of Black Walnut Green Hull Tincture and 1 tsp. of the ground Papaya seeds. Pierce three Caprylic acid capsules with a needle and squeeze them into your mixture. Mix rapidly again. Add 1 heaping tablespoon of Psyllium husk and 1 heaping tablespoon of Psyllium powder and mix rapidly. Drink it all down immediately, adding a little water between sips to keep the mixture liquidy and loose enough to drink.

Sure, it tastes a little gross and the texture is thick, but I guarantee you will be happily amazed by the results. Friends that I have introduced to this bang my door down when they run out of the ingredients, begging me for more.   Drinking 1-2 of these a day (I take one in morning and one before bed) is usually enough to start to see a huge difference in your health.

You will literally start to feel "clean on the inside", as hard as that feeling is to describe. Please, look up "Psyllium and Bentonite" on Google or Yahoo and see what other people are saying about this remedy. Those who start really get hooked on it.

One of the great benefits of this regimen is that it makes you feel so full, it is a fantastic dieting aid! The full feeling lasts for hours and hours. You may have to remind yourself to eat! And you will definitely eat less when you do sit down to a meal.

Another benefit is you will use less toilet paper :) I won't elaborate on that...you'll see what I mean soon enough.

One warning...take this at least an hour before or after you take any medications because the Bentonite and Diatomaceous earth will soak up the medicine as if it were toxins (which it is, but don't get me started on that). Those two ingredients adsorbe (leech out and bind with) toxins, parasites and foreign particles in your body, removing waste products from blood and tissues. You'll literally feel what I'm talking about.

Make sure you drink lots of water and juice and chemical-free beverages throughout the day to keep things moving.

I'll post more health protection methods in the near future.

Good luck, and please give this one a try. So many people I have introduced to this have thanked me again and again. I want you to feel as good as we do!

Back to plastic surgery. If you have your surgery in a location distant from your home you absolutely must stay at least 2 weeks! Please don't think that you can go out on a safari, splashing in the ocean or even lying in the sun. All of these activities are major no-no's!

Your plastic surgery vacation should be all about plastic surgery and not about vacation adventures. As always, **FOLLOW YOUR DOCTOR'S INSTRUCTIONS!** To err on the side of babying yourself is the best defense against complications and/or infection.

If you refuse to take responsibility for caring for yourself properly after your surgery, you will have no one to blame but yourself should you get infections or complications. Please do all you can to protect your health and your cosmetic surgery results.

It is my opinion that many doctors' reputations and practices have been damaged by patients who, out of ignorance or apathy, have not cared for themselves properly and/or followed their doctors' post-op instructions. This is a very unfortunate situation.

If a movement was created in the area of personal healthcare responsibility, I believe the burden on the medical community would be reduced, as well as the personal suffering of patients who neglect their own health until it is too late, and then want to point fingers at anyone and everyone they can. With the availability of quality information regarding hygiene and health on the internet, there is little excuse for not doing all you can to protect your own well-being.

Procedure Details...What You Can Expect Before, During and After Surgery

Rhinoplasty (Nose Job)

One of the most popular cosmetic surgery procedures is that of the "nose job". Indeed, a well-performed rhinoplasty can dramatically change a person's appearance. Usually, a surgeon will advise younger patients that it is best to wait until age 17 or older before undergoing this procedure, as it is preferred that the nose "finish growing" before augmentation. In rare instances, a surgeon will perform rhinoplasty on younger patients if the situation is so dire that it is worried that the child will suffer abuse or be ostracized by peers, doing irreparable emotional damage.

When performing rhinoplasty, transverse incisions are made inside of the nose, so that there is no visible external scar. Through these incisions, the surgeon shapes and models the nasal bones and cartilage to obtain the desired profile and/or narrowing. In rare occasions, it is necessary to make an additional incision at the level of the nostrils. Some surgeons prefer to perform the operation under general anesthesia, while others use only local anesthesia with sedation. On occasion, synthetic prostheses and internal grafts are used to give form, shape and support to the nasal pyramid. If there is respiratory difficulty, it may be necessary to modify the prosthesis or reshape the cartilage of the nasal partition.

Following the procedure, a nasal obstruction and plaster cast are usually placed. The duration of the wearing of the cast is relative to the individual situation and left to the discretion of the surgeon. Postoperative inflammation, swelling and bruising is to be expected and usually dissipates within the first two weeks post-op.

It is not possible to see the full results of the "nose job" until several months post-operatively. In some cases, additional intervention may be necessary to "tweak" the final rhinoplasty results.

Ideally, as with all cosmetic procedures, the end result is a nose that is harmonious with the entire facial aspect, as natural looking and unremarkable as possible. As most people would agree, they would rather hear the comment of, "You look great!" rather than, "Hey, I love your 'new' nose!"

The ultimate result depends on the degree of difficulty of the procedure (i.e. the magnitude and deformity of the original nose), the skill and experience of the surgeon and the opportunity for minor surgical adjustment in the postoperative phase.

Complications are rare with this type of surgery, however as mentioned above, there is sometimes need for minor adjustment following the main surgery.

Chin Enhancement/Implant

Retrusion of the chin is a fairly common facial aspect, and often accompanies the appearance of a large nose. For that reason, many patients undergo chin implant in addition to rhinoplasty, to give an overall "balance" to the profile. In some cases, a chin implant alone can make the nose look less protuberant. Increasing the pronouncement of the chin can create the illusion of a stronger facial character and give the patient a more confident, mature appearance.

Chin enhancement is achieved by means of fashioning and sliding forward a portion of bone from the jaw, or most frequently by means of insertion of a synthetic prosthesis. The procedure is performed under local or general anesthesia depending upon the personal preferences of both surgeon and patient.

Yet another technique is autologous fat transplantation, where the surgeon takes a sampling of fat from a donor region of the patient's body and implants it in the chin. This is a safer method that gets very good results.

The body may reabsorb some or all of the fat over a period of several years, so this procedure may need to be redone in time. However, it gives a very natural appearance and there is less likely to be any rejection or complication.

As in rhinoplasty, complications occur infrequently and may consist of displacement of implant, requiring subsequent relocation. Local infection is extremely rare.

Cheek Enhancement/Implant

A popular cosmetic procedure today is that of cheekbone enhancement or implant. This gives a very elegant, shapely appearance to the face that most ladies try to achieve with the daily application of blusher or rouge. Cheek enhancement lends a "sculpted" appearance to the face, making the face appear less wide and more angular...very supermodelesque.

Some plastic surgeons employ the insertion of synthetic prostheses, which are implanted to perfectly adapt to the surface of the malar bone. Prefabricated prostheses are available in the common suitable form, although some are made to be specially "carved" by the surgeon for a customized fit and dimension.

Still other cosmetic surgeons will resort to use an "organic weave" transplant formed from fibrous and/or adipose (fat) tissue taken directly from the patient. This type of procedure demands additional extraction from the patient, and is sometimes reduced in size over time due to resorption by the patient. In such cases, repetition of surgery is required.

The procedure is performed through incisions made on the inside of the mouth over the crease between the superior lip and upper jawbone. A tunnel is formed up to the desired area of placement, and the implant is inserted and situated.

If the procedure is performed in conjunction with rhytidectomy (face lift), the implants may be worked in from incisions performed for the facelift. When performed via the mouth, resulting scars are of course not visible.

Results are most frequently very satisfactory to the patient. Complications are extremely rare and consist mainly of sub optimal positioning or displacement requiring additional surgical intervention and replacement.

Even rarer are complications of local infection needing drainage, reduced sensitivity of the superior lip or decreased mobility. Should these complications arise, they usually resolve themselves within a few days or weeks following surgery.

Again, optimal results are those of a natural appearance.

Otoplasty (Ear Pinning)

Many children suffer from protruding ears, and subsequently grow up being teased and called names ("Dumbo", etc.) Although cosmetic surgery is ideally performed on no patient under the age of 16, otoplasty is an interventional procedure frequently performed on children, to save them the pain of being harassed by friends and classmates.

Cosmetic surgeons are usually willing to perform this surgery on children due to the fact that even though indications exist that the growth of the ears persists throughout life, by the age of 5 or 6 the ears are nearly the size that they will be in adulthood.

The procedure of otoplasty does not actually alter the "size" of the ears. Rather, an incision is made behind the ear, at which time the cosmetic surgeon remodels the cartilage of the ear, reducing the depth of the shell and removing leftover skin.

Most often, a bandage is placed that perfectly models all parts of the ear, allowing the incision to heal in proper position. It is advised that the ears remain taped in the correct position for two weeks post-operatively.

The results of otoplasty are permanent. There should not be need for readjustment later in life. Complications are rare, mainly including local infection of incision or need for minor aesthetic surgical adjustments.

Rhytidectomy (Face Lift)

Facelift is a general term applied to diverse procedures to elevate the facial structures and tighten the facial skin, with the main objective of reducing wrinkles and giving an overall more youthful appearance.

The bony structure of the face, heredity factors and cutaneous texture all play important roles in the final outcome of the rhytidectomy.

The 'face lift' usually involves the area of the neck, 'jowls' or sagging skin of the jaw area, cheeks, perioral (area round the mouth), periorbital (area around the eyes) and forehead. Sometimes the adjustment of the area of the forehead and eyebrows must be done as separate procedures depending upon the existing skin turgor (or laxity).

Face lift incisions are made on the inside of the hairline, through the existing skin folds in front of the ears, continuing behind the ear and following the natural hairline. In many instances, the incisions are extended through subcutaneous tissues and into the muscular tissue. Flaccid muscles of the face are then sutured and "tightened", as are the layers of skin and subcutaneous tissue. This gives the entire face an overall "firmer" appearance.

Following surgery, there is normally quite a bit of swelling and bruising, sensation of facial tenseness and possibly some sponginess of some areas of the face and neck. Within two to four weeks, these sensations will dissipate and the bruising will heal. Most of the scarring will be hidden within the natural hairline and normal skin folds around the ears. Scars behind the ears can be easily hidden with an appropriate hairstyle.

The patient should not expect to be able to wash or brush hair for quite some time…some surgeons advise waiting at least one month. It is also usually recommended that the patient avoid sun exposure and to use sunscreen and hydrating lotions to keep the skin moist.

It is no longer advised that a patient wait until 60 to 70 years of age before undergoing rhytidectomy. In fact, many surgeons recommend getting "mini- face lifts" starting as early as the 40's.

Good results are much easier to achieve and maintain if smaller procedures are performed as "preventative measures", before the face looses muscular turgor and the skin becomes thin and flaccid. It is much easier to maintain a youthful appearance than it is to regain a youthful appearance!

In expert hands, complications resulting from this procedure are very few and mostly transitory, i.e. hematoma, defects of healing, cutaneous injuries, loss of hair at scar areas, altered motility of eyebrows or lips, numbness, tingling and loss of sensation in the face, as well as local infection of the incision lines. Risks associated with the procedure are statistically rare, and are widely compensated by the positive result of the surgery.

Blepharoplasty (Aesthetic Surgical Fixation of the Eyelids)

Some of the first signs of aging occur in the eye area. Although there are many creams and lotions on the market that claim to slow this process, there is no real cure for drooping eyebrows, crows' feet and sagging upper eyelids as well as under-eye "bags", other than surgical intervention.

In some cases, the condition is clearly due to familial tendency (heredity), and in these cases decline of the eye area can occur at a fairly early age.

Environmental pollution, smoking, extreme and frequent sun exposure, poor nutrition, stress, chronic insomnia and habitual rubbing or tugging of the eye area can also cause the aforementioned condition.

Blepharoplasty can be performed as an isolated procedure but often is performed as part of an accompanying surgery, most generally in association with rhytidectomy. Depending upon this, and the preferences of the surgeon, the surgical intervention will be made under local anesthesia with sedation or general anesthesia.

Under the skin and orbicular muscle (muscles surrounding the eye) exist compartments that contain fat. This fat is surgically reduced/ removed to eliminate the appearance of "bags".

Depending on the muscular tension of the eyelids, the surgeon may also surgically fix orbicular muscles, thus restoring normal youthful muscle tension in the orbicular area.

Incisions in the upper eyelids are made in the natural crease lines, thus minimizing any visible scarring. Excess skin is removed when suitable, as well as excess fatty deposits. Incisions in the lower lids are made inferior and very close to the eyelash line.

Immediately following the procedure, the patient's eyes will usually be covered with moist gauze dressings, which will remain for a day. The sutures commonly are covered with surgical tape for the first few days (3-4 days).

There is usually some bruising associated, especially if the patient has lower eyelid surgery. There will be a week or two of "black eyes". The upper lids may show some swelling and bruising as well for a week or two. Stitches generally remain in for 7-10 days.

You will most likely look like a prizefighter for a while following blepharoplasty, and will want to keep your dark glasses handy for public outings. This is both cosmetic and medical in purpose, as it is not uncommon to have a bit of intolerance to light for a couple of weeks.

Other possible minor irritations and discomforts following this surgery are hematoma and subconjunctival conjunctivitis (blood collections under the eyelids or in the eyeball itself). These resolve themselves on their own or with suitable medical treatment (eyedrops).

Sometimes during the first days or weeks following surgery, the patient may not be able to totally close the eyelids, mainly during sleep. This is normal; the orbicular muscles recover their normal tone on their own, possibly helped along with appropriate exercises.

Because of the increased field of vision that many patients experience following this type of surgery, there is a bit of an adjustment period necessary (again, roughly 2-3 weeks to feel "comfortable"). The scars that can be visible are normally fine reddened or purplish lines that resolve themselves within several weeks of surgery.

Several additional techniques exist, including the utilization of laser therapy to reduce crow's feet, in particular. The result of this surgical intervention is very favorable and lasting, and in general the bags of the eyelids do not usually reappear.

Contour Threads

One of the most exciting developments in the area of facial rejuvenation is the use of the patented and now FDA-approved Contour Threads [TM]. In a minimally invasive procedure, these little "barbed" strings are tunneled down through the facial skin and then pulled up, which opens the little thorny spines which line the edges of the threads and grab the surrounding tissues. Sagging cheeks, brows and jawlines are then pulled up, and the Contour Threads [TM] are anchored in place somewhere along the hairline, resulting in an instantly younger, tighter appearance of the face.

Because of the tiny incisions where the threads are introduced, scaring is minimal. The threads are made of clear polypropylene, which has been used as a component in various surgical implant devices and materials for years.

Best of all, results are usually permanent because your body will naturally regenerate collagen around the sutures, permanently "fixing" the results in place.

Contour Threads [TM] are not for everyone, however. Results are best for those whose faces are just starting to droop. Over-pulling of too much excess skin will just form deeper creases in a different area (an accordion effect).

The procedure is quite safe and non-invasive, and recovery time ranges from 1-7 days. As mentioned above, results are usually visible immediately after surgery. However, some swelling and a little bruising is possible.

Like all cosmetic surgery procedures, there is risk for potential complications including but not limited to: hematoma (formation of blood pools below the skin), seroma (formation of serous fluid pockets below the skin), infection, swelling, asymmetry, bleeding, pigmentation (discoloration of the skin), palpable threads (being able to "feel" the threads below the skin), puckering of skin, skin feeling too tight, numbness/facial nerve damage, and migration or breaking of the threads themselves.

Chemical Peel

Laxity of the facial skin that occurs with age, including deep facial lines, crevices and drooping can only be reversed through face lift or face "stretching".

However, facelift is not so effective for fine lines and wrinkles, in which case the treatments of choice are commonly the "Chemical Peel", dermabrasion or laser surgery.

In all three of these treatments, the goal is the removal or ablation of the superficial layer of skin so that the fine, small wrinkles of the face are diminished or eliminated thus restoring the skin's smoothness.

Additionally these procedures may serve to correct superficial scars, depressions, or cutaneous irregularity (such as resulting from chicken pox or acne), spots or hyperkeratosis. In some instances, the procedures of chemical dermabrasion and peeling can be combined.

In the case of chemical peeling, a chemical solution (most commonly Phenol or trichloroacetic acid [TCA]) is applied to those areas of the face that are to be treated. The solution can be applied to the entire face, or simply to specific areas such as the regions surrounding the mouth and/or cheeks.

The entire procedure is performed within 1-2 hours, and normally is performed without anesthesia, although sedation and EKG monitoring may be utilized in certain situations. Although chemical peels are usually performed on an outpatient basis, a full-facial Phenol peel may require 1-2 days of hospitalization.

The type of dressing that is applied to the skin following such procedures depends on the nature of the procedure and the surgeon's personal preference.

Following any of these procedures, the face will appear "raw"…very red indeed. Either type of chemical solution could cause transitory and temporary throbbing, tingling, swelling, redness, and acute sensitivity to sun.

In the case of a Phenol peel there is the chance of long lasting (perhaps permanent) lightening of the skin in the area treated, with the possibility of permanent inability of the skin to tan.

Additional complications that may ensue include the development of whiteheads (temporary), infection, scarring, flare-up of skin allergies, blistering, or development of cold sores. Phenol chemical peels may result in abnormal permanent change of skin color and rarely causes heart rhythm irregularities.

Generally, a protective scab forms that will be shed as the layers of skin beneath it regenerate.

Once this scab has fallen off (generally new skin forms within 7-21 days with Phenol, 5-10 days with TCA), the new layer of epidermis, very pink in color, will have replaced the superior layer of the skin…the layer that formerly showed fine lines and wrinkles.

The pink color will dissipate gradually with the course of time and it is possible to disguise this somewhat with foundation makeup after about 2 or 3 weeks post-procedure.

In the 5-7 days immediately following the procedure there will almost certainly be swelling of varying degrees.

The surgeon will certainly recommend that the patient avoid any kind of sun exposure until the skin recovers it's epidermal layer, and thus normal resistance to weather conditions. Premature sun exposure can produce areas of cutaneous discoloration that could require additional peeling in the future.

During the postoperative period, it is advisable to use a sunscreen lotion with a very high SPF.

Patients can generally return to normal activities within 2-4 weeks, and can expect complete healing and dissipation of facial redness within 3-6 months.

As in other procedures, the result will depend to a large extent on the quality of the skin prior to surgery.

The result of chemical peel and dermabrasion is normally very satisfactory, although the postoperative period can be difficult due to the high degree of facial discoloration.

In many cases, the procedure will need to be repeated every several years. Chemical peeling and dermabrasion may not be a "permanent fix".

Dermabrasion obtains a similar effect as chemical peel, but instead of using a chemical solution to "dissolve" the superficial skin layers, the skin is "buffed" with a sandpaper-like device attached to a rotary wheel.

Facial dermabrasion may take anywhere from just several minutes to 1 hour, although more than one treatment may be required.

This procedure is performed under local anesthesia, numbing spray or in rare cases, general anesthesia and usually on an outpatient basis.

Patients can expect to experience post-procedure tingling, burning, itching, slight swelling and transitory redness. There most likely will be lightening of treated skin, acute sensitivity to sun, as well as loss of ability to tan.

Possible complications are the same as those of a chemical peel.

Getting back to work should take about 2 weeks, not resuming strenuous activities for 4-6 weeks. The redness should fade completely in about 3 months postoperatively. Return of pigmentation/sun exposure in 6 to 12 months. The results are often permanent, although new wrinkles may form as skin ages.

In the case of laser dermabrasion, a CO2 laser is used to "vaporize" or burn away the outer layers of the facial skin. All indications of laser facial resurfacing are similar to those of dermabrasion.

Botox Injection (Botulinium Toxin)

Botox Injection is currently the method of choice among men and women who wish to reduce facial lines with the minimum of intervention.

Botox (a derivative of the Botulinium Toxin) is injected into muscular areas of the face that experience the most tension, thus causing facial lines and creases. Such areas commonly include the forehead, between the eyebrows and near the corners of the eyes where "crow's feet" develop.

The Botox causes a paralysis to the muscle tissue in these areas, typically lasting up to 6 months in duration, but more commonly lasting only 2-4 months. Most patients get repeat treatments every 3 months.

Discomfort caused by the injections is usually mild stinging accompanied by a little swelling on occasion. This usually subsides within 4-24 hours following injection. Infrequently, a patient will develop drooping of the eyebrow or eyelid lasting up to a few weeks.

The desired results of Botox injection are not apparent until 2-4 days following administration.

BODY CONTOURING

Grouped under the concept of "Body Contouring" are many different procedures, which modify the volume of various regions of the body.

Breast augmentation, breast reduction, breast lifting, liposuction/liposculpture of the arms, back, abdomen, flanks, hips and thighs, as well as gluteal augmentation (buttock lifting), thigh lift and arm lift all fall under the category of Body Contouring.

While some of these procedures leave the patient only small scars, which are difficult to detect with the human eye, others inevitably by their nature leave long scars, which may be difficult to hide under certain clothing.

The plastic surgeon should, of course, take great care and do everything within his power to obtain only the finest scar. Nevertheless, the final quality of a scar is strongly influenced by personal characteristics of healing, differing from patient to patient.

The best the surgeon can do is to instruct the patient in proper wound care and place the incisions in the best naturally less visible areas of the body. Unfortunately, at the present time it is not possible to completely erase them. Scars are by their nature the price that one may have to pay for a more pleasing figure through plastic surgery.

Mammoplasty (Breast Augmentation)

In this procedure, the surgeon places implants or mammary prostheses behind the existing mammary glands of the breasts. The positioning of these implants can be made behind the pectoral muscle.

The surgeon should evaluate the advantages and disadvantages of each technique on a per patient basis, and explain to the patient which method is preferable.

In order to place the prostheses, the surgeon may use one of several different approaches including through an incision in the axillary area (armpit), through an incision around the areola (nipple) known as circumareolar, at the level of the breast crease (beneath the breast), or most recently through a tunnel created through the upper abdomen originating in a small incision in the navel (bellybutton) known as infraumbilical incision.

The prosthesis itself consists of a circular "bag" filled with silicone gel, saline serum (saltwater), or both in different compartments. The bag itself is made of a synthetic material, usually silicone.

Breast augmentation surgery is commonly performed under epidural or local anesthesia with sedation, and is completed within 1-2 hours.

The type of bandage used post-operatively will vary according to the surgeon's preference.

The patient should be able to return to work within 3-4 days. The incisions are normally quite small and difficult to detect.

Postoperatively, some surgeons may recommend massage to the area to avoid retraction of the capsule that the body forms around the prosthesis, although other surgeons prefer a period of prolonged immobilization of the breast region.

The most frequent complication of mammoplasty is increase of the capsular retraction (contractural). In this instance, the body surrounds the prosthesis with a fibrous layer of tissue that may become thickened and unnaturally firm.

The cause of this complication is not clearly defined, and occurs in approximately 10% of patients who undergo breast augmentation.

In the case that this complication develops, the surgeon should indicate which measures are appropriate to correct the situation including the possibility of breaking the capsule by external maneuvers or further surgical intervention.

Other possible local complications include hematoma, infection, and intolerance of sutures or prostheses that would require appropriate medical or surgical treatment. The incidence of such complications is not frequent.

Following the procedure, the patient will undoubtedly suffer quite a bit of chest discomfort for a minimum of 2 weeks post-op. Bruising and swelling are also to be expected.

Breast Reduction (Gynecomastia – Male or Female)

The reduction of the breasts is quite a bit more complicated than the enlargement of the breasts. During the surgery, the surgeon will most likely have to reduce the areola (nipple) to a more suitable size and replace it in a more correct location.

Although the techniques of breast reduction surgery are diverse, most often it requires circumareolar incisions, vertical incisions and oblique horizontal incisions, or incisions in the natural mammary folds.

Commonly performed under epidural or general anesthesia, this procedure requires hospitalization of 24-48 hours.

The suture lines must be made with great meticulous care to obtain the shortest and finest of scars possible.

Again, considerable scarring is to be expected due to the nature of the procedure, with the most visible scars being those of the submammary furrow (beneath the breasts). In time, these scars usually diminish considerably in visibility.

In some patients who experience more extensive scarring, it is advisable to undergo scar revision approximately 6 months post-operatively, which can be done under local anesthesia and sedation.

During the intervention, the surgeon sculpts down the skin, mammary gland and excessive fat and relocates the areola in its correct location, remodeling the breast accordingly.

Following the procedure, the surgeon usually will place his or her preferred type of bandage/dressing. The patient should expect bruising and swelling in the postoperative period. Possible complications include risk of reduction or total loss of sensitivity of the areolae. Most patients will experience this, only to regain sensation in the area over time.

In rare cases, there may be some fatty necrosis (fatty tissue death), wound dehiscence (oozing) or partial or total loss of the areola. In the case of areola necrosis or detachment, the area would be cosmetically repaired by means of an appropriate tissue graft/prosthesis. This complication is very rare, but the patient should be informed of the possibility.

For men, this procedure is usually more of a simple liposuction combined with trimming of excess skin and suturing.

Mastopexy (Breast Lift)

Similar to the breast reduction procedure, a breast lift improves the appearance of flaccid or pendulous breasts.

The surgeon may remodel the breasts in the same manner as discussed in the explanation of the breast reduction surgery. In other cases, prostheses may be an easier and more appropriate option. In this case, prostheses are inserted mainly to restore the projection of the breasts, rather than to make them larger.

Recovery time and scarring are similar to that of breast reduction. The entire procedure is performed within 1-3 hours on an outpatient basis, and is performed on an inpatient or outpatient basis depending upon the individual situation.

Results are generally favorable and long lasting, but can be negatively influenced by pregnancy, aging and/or excessive weight loss or gain.

Abdominoplasty (Tummy Tuck)

A tummy tuck is a procedure whereby a horizontal incision is made in a "French bikini" line across the lower abdomen and just superior to the pubic hairline extending from hip to hip.

The incision is much similar to that of a Cesarean section. Usually, this is used in combination with liposuction, both suctioning and excising (cutting out) layers of fat from the lower and sometimes upper abdomen.

The surgery is done under general or epidural anesthesia.

Most surgeons "tighten" the stomach muscles themselves using sutures in a corset fashion. Several inches of skin and flab from the lower abdomen are removed, usually including removal of most stretch marks.

The incision is closed and a new "belly button" is created by means of a circular incision in the area where the original navel had been and suturing the edges in place. When done with care, the new "belly button" looks just like the original once the wound heals. The circumferential scar is usually very fine and not at all noticeable if done with care.

The entire surgical procedure takes between 2-5 hours.

Immediately following surgery, when the patient awakens from anesthesia, she or he will be helped out of bed. The patient will not be able to stand up straight, as the muscles and skin of the stomach have been surgically "shortened".

It will take time, usually several days, for the patient to be able to walk fully upright. The patient will be very bent over when standing in the initial hours and days after surgery, but this is a situation that gradually rectifies itself as the abdomen realizes its new form and the body adjusts.

Significant pain is not uncommon, but is usually short in duration, lasting only 3-4 days. For most patients, the pain is a feeling like having done 250 sit-ups in an "out of shape" physical condition.

Coughing, laughter and rolling over in bed can cause significant pain. The patient should definitely have a friend, family member or home health aide available for at least a week after surgery to help with getting out of bed, using the toilet, etc.

A compression garment, or elastic girdle, is put on the patient immediately following closure in the operating room. This girdle is to be worn for a minimum of one month following surgery, preferably six weeks.

The patient will need to stay in the hospital following surgery for 24-48 hours

Although the incision in the lower abdomen is long, extending from hipbone to hipbone, if it is done with precision and care it is easily hidden beneath normal bikini underwear or bikini bathing suit. There is normally no need to wear brief style underwear or one-piece bathing suit.

However, it can take up to a year for the scar to fade to the patient's liking.

The result is a taught, smooth, flat abdomen. With the exception of subsequent pregnancy, the results are long lasting and patients are usually very pleased with their new waistlines and flat tummies.

There is almost always some degree of swelling following surgery, but this usually fully dissipates within 3-6 months. There is always numbness of the abdomen to varying degrees, often lasting up to 6 months or a little longer.

In cases of moderate to severe obesity, the patient may need to go back in for a little additional liposuction after about 6 months to remove any superficial fat that was missed at surgery.

A tummy tuck is major abdominal surgery including superficial, subdermal and muscular incisions and suturing. For this reason, the patient should plan on a recovery period of 3-4 weeks, only the first week or so of that being full bed rest.

Even during the first week, it is important that the patient gets out of bed several times a day and walks for a tolerable period of time to avoid complications of unwanted blood clotting (deep venous thrombosis). It is important for the patient to understand that superior self-care in both the pre- and post-surgical period is vital. Sutures will be removed in 7-10 days after surgery.

If the patient plans to have children, it is not advisable to have a tummy tuck until after all desired pregnancies.

As in all cases, the degree of scarring varies from patient to patient. Should the scar be too unsightly and unacceptable to the patient, it is possible to revise the scar following one year post-operatively.

Though rare, possible complications include a zone of loss of sensation or vitality (necrosis) of the abdomen, seroma requiring aspiration (suction).

Liposuction/Lipoaspiration/ Liposculpture/Suction-Assisted Lipectomy

Liposuction, the surgical "vacuum" removal of fat from the body, although not a recommended form of weight reduction is an excellent solution for those with unsightly fatty deposits, bulges and "rolls" that are resistant to diet and exercise.

The technique consists essentially of the aspiration (suctioning) of the fat of a particular area of the body. A blunt cannula (hollow needle), which is attached to a suctioning machine, is introduced through a very small incision in the skin. The cannula is tunneled through the skin repeatedly, suctioning more fat with each pass.

The miniscule size of the incision necessary to allow passage of the cannula is perhaps one of the most favorable aspects of this particular cosmetic procedure, usually being no longer than 10 mm.

In addition, the incision does not need to be in the exact area of the planned reduction, thus allowing the surgeon to place the incision in a much less visible place on the body.

Several forms of liposuction exist, including tumescent liposuction and ultrasound-assisted lipoplasty.

The tumescent liposuction technique consists of infusing the fat cells with a combination of saline solution and local anesthetic prior to liposuction, which reduces postoperative bruising and swelling.

This type of liposuction is usually performed in the areas of the chin, cheeks, neck, upper arms, hips, thighs, and knees, above breasts, abdomen, buttocks, calves or ankles.

To facilitate the removal of large amounts of fat, and for areas of the body, which are more fibrous in nature, the method of ultrasound-assisted lipoplasty is sometimes used.

An ultrasound instrument is inserted beneath the skin, "liquefying" the fat before it is suctioned out through the cannula.

Most liposuction procedures are performed within 1 to 2 hours or more, ultrasound-assisted techniques taking 20-40 percent longer than traditional liposuction.

Anesthesia used may be local, epidural, or general depending upon the extent and area of the surgery, usually outpatient. Procedures that are more extensive may require a brief hospital stay.

The patient will definitely suffer some temporary bruising, swelling, numbness, soreness and/or burning sensation. Those who undergo the tumescent technique will have temporary fluid drainage from incision sites.

Slightly larger incisions may need to be made to accommodate ultrasound-assisted liposuction.

Possible complications could include asymmetry, sagging of skin, uneven or "dimpled" appearance, pigmentation changes, injury to skin and surrounding tissues, severe fluid retention, excessive fluid and/or shock, infection of incision sites or involved tissue. The heat generated by the ultrasound device has caused burns in rare cases.

All of these complications are quite rare.

Liposuction patients may return to work within 1 to 2 weeks, with more strenuous activity within 2 to 4 weeks. Recovery from swelling and bruising will take 1-6 months or more. Use of tumescent technique or UAL may decrease post-operative bruising and swelling.

Results are permanent, although patients may still gain weight in areas where fat was not suctioned.

The main variable that determines the results obtained from liposuction is the original skin elasticity of the patient. If the skin is excessively flaccid, liposuction may result in a saggy "deflated" appearance. In this case, it is often recommended that the patient have the appropriate "lift" procedure for the area of skin flaccidity (sagging, i.e. thigh lift, upper arm lift, etc.)

Thigh Lift

Following major weight loss, it is common for the skin of the thighs, especially the inner thigh, to become extremely loose and unsightly. To remedy the appearance of this sagging, a thigh lift procedure may be the only suitable option.

In a thigh lift, incisions are made over the upper-inner thigh and in some cases around into the crease below the buttocks area. The skin is pulled up, excess trimmed off and edges sutured. The surgery is often performed in conjunction with liposuction of the thighs. The resulting suture line is quite well hidden in the groin crease when performed with care.

The patient can expect to be very uncomfortable for at least 2 weeks following surgery and will need assistance with getting around and using the bathroom. It is important, because of location, to pay special attention to wound cleaning and care.

The patient can expect swelling and bruising for up to 3-4 weeks post-operatively, as well as a very "tight" feeling in the thighs. Walking and sitting will be uncomfortable for a few weeks. Stitches should be removed within 7-10 days. The patient will not be able to work or drive for a minimum of two weeks, with no exercise for at least 4 weeks.

Brachioplasty (Arm Lift)

In order to tighten loose, flabby skin that hangs beneath the upper arms ("batwings"), a brachioplasty is performed. In this procedure, a long incision is made in a "T-shape", with the cross of the T being made in the crease of the armpit and the rest of the incision being made lengthwise from the armpit to the elbow.

Fat is removed surgically and/or with liposuction and the incisions are closed, following drain placement. The drain will exit near the elbow.

The patient will be placed in bandages and a compression garment. Stitches will be removed in 7-10 days, along with the drain removal.

The patient can expect to be extremely uncomfortable for at least 3 weeks. It is very important that the patient does not lift or raise the arms. Assistance with daily chores including bathing and hair brushing will be necessary for approximately 2 weeks.

Because of the placement of the suture lines, it is very important that the patient pay extra care to wound care and cleaning. The patient will not be able to raise arms or do any lifting for at least a month, preferably 6 weeks.

Buttock Augmentation

Enhancement of the gluteal area (butt, buttocks) is performed using either solid silicone implants or autologous fat (fat removed from other areas of the patient). The solid silicone implants used in this procedure are very dense and much more resistant to rupture than those used for breast augmentation.

Ideally, the incisions are made on the inner crease of the buttocks, so scars are not visible. If there is worry of impending infection, however, the incisions may be placed in the crease where the upper thighs meet the buttocks.

The implants are inserted into a cavity that the surgeon has previously created separating superficial tissues/fascia (fibrous tissue) from the muscle below. The implants are positioned so that the patient will not actually be sitting "on" the implants...more in the area of the pockets of your jeans lay.

If the autologous fat implantation method is used, fat is harvested from areas of the body where there is an overabundance of fat (belly, hips, etc.), then implanted into the buttocks.

General anesthesia is most often used during this procedure. Recovery time is two weeks or more, during which the patient will have to spend most of the time lying on her/his stomach. Swelling and bruising is to be expected.

Sutures will be removed 10 days postoperatively. It is important that the patient moves extremely slowly and avoids sitting for at least 2 weeks.

Vaginal Remodeling

One of the most controversial areas of plastic surgery being performed currently is that of vaginal plastic surgery. Taboo as this may seem, many women have suffered from the ravages of childbirth in silence. The advent of laser technology coupled with a more honest and liberated society have brought solutions for this often troublesome situation. Just as with the rest of the body, genital tissues lose their turgor over time. There is no way to know how many love lives have been altered or ruined by this physical phenomenon. It is definitely an issue that is kept as secret as possible.

Laser Vaginal Rejuvenation ® is more of a gynecological surgical procedure than cosmetic or plastic surgery per se, but I wanted to mention it here for those who are in need of its benefits. For those seeking corrective vaginal surgery, either for enhanced sexual functioning or urinary prolapse, I highly recommend that you visit **http://www.serulle.com**, the web site of Dominican Republic gynecological surgeon Dr. Yuseff Serulle, or contact him by phone at: (809) 336-2544. Dr. Serulle's web site is highly informative regarding various vaginal remodeling/rejuvenation procedures.

Hair Transplantation (mini or micro-hair grafting)

In hair transplantation, a strip of hair is surgically excised from back/lower region of the scalp (donating area) and is observed under a special microscope to visualize the structures of the hair and to separate them in groups of one, two, three or four hairs with its intact bulb (follicular units).

These hairs are then individually inserted into the area of baldness with careful precision to orient the hairs in a direction compatible with natural growth patterns. The procedure can last between 2-6 hours depending on the extent of the bald zone to re-populated with the "donor" hairs.

During the procedure the patient remains wide-awake, relaxed and without pain. Immediately following the completion of the procedure, the patient is able to leave the clinic.

The recovery period is usually 2-3 weeks in duration, during which time the patient will experience some scabbing and perhaps swelling and tingling of the area treated. The patient is usually allowed to wear a loose-fitting cap or hat during the recovery period, depending upon the extent and location of the surgical area.

The hair usually shows signs of growth in about 21 days following surgery. Once healing is complete and the hair is growing normally, it can be washed and trimmed as necessary.

Results are normally permanent, since the donor hairs are taken from an area of the scalp that rarely goes through natural hair loss.

Bariatric Surgery

Although bariatric surgery (a.k.a. weight loss surgery) is not considered plastic surgery, I have chosen to include it here at the request of many of my past readers. A good percentage of the readers of **"How to Get High-Quality Plastic Surgery…CHEAP!"** have already undergone either lap banding or stomach bypass procedures and are now in need of many plastic surgery procedures to tighten loose skin they now have as a result of their massive weight loss. They are, of course, also curious to find out if bariatric surgery is available at a lower cost in the Dominican Republic.

According to the American Heart Association, the number of Americans who are obese has increased over 75% since 1991. A well-publicized statistic acknowledges that sixty-four percent of the U.S. population is overweight or obese, according to the Centers for Disease Control and Prevention. Thusly, it is estimated that over 400,000 deaths in America each year are due in part to the condition of being overweight/obese. Bariatric surgery has become a necessary solution for those whose weight gain has become out of control, and who are at least 100 pounds overweight or have a Body Mass Index of 40 or higher.

The average cost of bariatric surgery in the United States is anywhere from $30,000-$70,000.00. In the Dominican Republic, it is usually around $10,000.00. As you can see, there is a huge savings. However, bariatric surgery does usually require a longer follow-up and recovery period than any plastic surgery procedure, so one would have to consider the cost (in both time and money) of staying in the Dominican Republic for up to 2 months following their surgery, then returning for a few days every 3-6 months for follow-up with the surgeon.

For the right people with the right attitude, this is an excellent solution. It is especially suitable for those who are able to work over the internet, as many of us are lucky enough to arrange in our modern society.

Below are descriptions of the available procedures, as well as insight into reasonable recovery times, results to expect and advice regarding what you may expect to encounter during your recovery.

Lap Band® (Adjustable Gastric Band)

In this procedure, an adjustable band made of silicone is placed laparoscopically around the upper part of the stomach. The band simply restricts the amount of food that can enter the stomach, thusly making the patient unable to eat beyond the amount that this now smaller stomach pouch can hold. This procedure is minimally invasive, and does not affect the absorption of nutrients, nor does it involved the dissection or stapling of any of the intestinal organs. The band is placed about 1.0 centimeter below the gastroesophageal junction. A port is placed in the skin, so that the band can be adjusted to rhythmically control weight loss progression.

This option is best for those who are minimally obese, and do not have a serious psychological over-eating disorder. Weight loss in this case is easily sabotaged with the eating of sweets and calorie-dense foods.

Loss of the total amount of excess weight is usually between 50-60%. This operation is not recommended for super-obese patients or those who habitually overeat and show lack of interest or ability to improve health habits.

Possible complications include migration or dislocation of the Lap-Band®, as well as local infection of the port site. In 1% of the cases, the Lap-Band® is not tolerated internally or causes digestive distress and must be removed or replaced.

Overeating may cause prolapse of the stomach, creating a larger pouch, in which case reoperation may be indicated. Various other complications are possible, including leakage of the saline fluid that inflates the Lap-Band®, reservoir or tubing problems. Your doctor should educate you regarding all possible complications and their inherent risks prior to your procedure.

Most patients return to full normal activity within 6 weeks following their surgery. However, this depends on the individual patient's state of health. Your doctor will coach you regarding nutritional and dietary changes, as well as any nutritional supplementation necessary to prevent untoward malnutrition following surgery.

Laparoscopic Gastric Bypass (Roux-en-Y)

Roux-en-Y, or gastric bypass surgery is the oldest of the bariatric surgery procedures, having been performed for approximately 34 years. In this procedure, food intake is restricted as well as causing malabsorption of food matter in the intestinal tract, meaning an inability of the body to fully digest the food and eventually turn it into fat.

During this operation, the surgeon staples off a large section of the stomach, creating a smaller pouch. As a result of the surgery, most of the stomach and part of the small intestine are bypassed, prohibiting absorption of food (and thusly calories) into the bloodstream.

Possible complications arising from Roux-en-Y are stenosis (scarring of the connection between the stomach and the intestine) which may induce vomiting, adhesions, leakage of intestinal fluid into the abdominal cavity immediately following surgery (occurs in less than 1%), and vitamin insufficiency (which can be treated orally with supplementation).

This procedure is good for those who overeat or are super-obese. Resulting weight loss is usually optimal, up to about 75% of the total excess weight. Weight loss is fairly rapid in the first few months following surgery, but may slow progressively.

Most patients return to full normal activity within 6 weeks following their surgery. However, this depends on the individual patient's state of health. Your doctor will coach you regarding nutritional and dietary changes, as well as any nutritional supplementation necessary to prevent untoward malnutrition following surgery.

Plastic Surgery Following Bariatric Surgery

In almost every case, post-bariatric surgery patients will find themselves needing some type of plastic surgery procedures to readjust their overstretched skin to their new, smaller body shape.

Usually, patients will need abdominoplasty (tummy tuck), brachioplasty (upper arm lift), buttock lift, face/neck lift, or a combination of any of the above. This, of course, depends upon the age of the patient, the number of years the patient was overweight prior to their bariatric surgery, as well as factors both genetic and lifestyle related. Those who are dedicated to a good exercise regimen throughout their post-bariatric surgery period are less likely to require major plastic surgery than those who don't exercise.

The cost of a major amount of plastic surgery "tucking" following weight loss surgery, where a patient has lost 100 lbs. or more, can cost up to $50,000.00…more in some Metropolitan areas. This on top of the $30,000-$70,000.00 that the patient spent on the initial weight loss surgery can put a truly satisfactory body size and shape out of reach for most people.

Choosing to have your surgery in the Dominican Republic will save you 40-60%! I will let you do the math. Another benefit of having your surgery performed in the Dominican Republic is the low cost of excellent aftercare that will be available to you. La Simetria has made it affordable to have on-call care of a licensed physician, 24-hours a day…something that is virtually unobtainable to the average middle-income American. And even if you don't choose a La Simetria vacation, your surgeon will most definitely be more accessible to you than if you were to have had your surgery in the U.S.

How to Prepare Yourself for Cosmetic Surgery in the Dominican Republic (or Anywhere Else!)

It is always advised that you enter into any surgery with a clear mind, a good attitude and a healthy body. I suggest following the Parasite Cleanse, Bowel Cleanse, Liver Cleanse and Kidney Cleanse as suggested by Dr. Hulda Clark in her book, **"The Cure for All Diseases"**.

All of these programs are accessible for free via the Internet at various web sites, including **http://www.Curezone.com**.

I highly recommend the above regimens to "do a little house cleaning" prior to your surgery. It is very important to try to rid your body of pathogens that may be laying dormant, waiting to take over when your body is in a weakened state, prior to any surgical or dental procedure, to reduce the risk of wound infection. It is only logical that the healthier you are going into surgery, the healthier you will be after your surgery.

Another herbal remedy that I have used to speed and ease recovery following surgery is Arnica Montana (30c or 30x), to start one week prior to surgery and continue up to three weeks following surgery.

The Arnica gel and massage oil are great, too…but don't use those until your wound is completely closed (2-3 weeks post-op).

This natural remedy greatly reduces pain, swelling and bruising and can be used to ease the symptoms of trauma in any situation. I highly recommend keeping some around the house at all times!

Also Bromelain, a homeopathic remedy derived from pineapple is helpful in this regard. Eating pineapple and drinking pineapple juice are also a good source of Bromelain as opposed to the pill form.

Good nutrition is very important prior to and after surgery, but then again, it always is! Make sure you're getting enough vitamins in your foods with lots of green leafy vegetables.

Do not take Ibuprofen or aspirin, and preferably have no caffeine two weeks pre- and post- surgery.

I suggest taking three basic amino acids: L-Lysine, L-Ornithine, and L-Arginine. L-Ornithine is especially helpful at night to promote deep and comfortable sleep. These help your tissues heal quicker, as amino acids are the building blocks of proteins.

Do not eat salt 2-3 weeks before and after surgery.

Exercise is always almost always good for the body. It is especially good to be physically strong prior to surgery. If you are uncomfortable with strenuous exercise, try some light weight lifting and Yoga. However, ask your doctor how long you should wait before resuming any exercise routine following your surgery.
I suggest you begin an exercise program (with a doctor's permission of course) prior to your surgery not only for the weight loss and

strengthening aspects, but because it is a good way for you to reconnect with your body.

It sounds kind of stupid, but most of us (especially those of us who want to change our bodies) ignore our bodies except to be critical of them. It is important that you mentally and spiritually care for your body to get you into the proper mentality for your transformation and proper healing.

Get yourself mentally and spiritually ready for your surgery. Surgery, especially cosmetic surgery, can take a toll on you emotionally.

It's a little scary to undergo any surgery, and there are undoubtedly a lot of feelings of excitement and hope mixed in. I highly recommend **Holosync** meditation CD's as a great help in reducing stress before your surgery and after.

Another program that is invaluable for overcoming stress, anxiety, enhancing emotional intelligence and helping with anger management is **The Sedona Method**, which is very comprehensive and really can straighten you out for good!

Recently, I discovered Dr. Laura DiGiorgio's subliminal CD's **"Preparation for Surgery"** and **"Accelerated Healing After Surgery"**. These special subliminal recordings ease the deep mental tension some people experience prior to surgery and silently coach your mind and body into healing at an accelerated rate.

Dr. DiGiorgio's subliminal recordings are PHENOMENAL! I use them all day, every day. They have helped me tremendously. In fact, I am listening to one right now as I write this!

She has a wide array of CD's that train your brain to improve your health, emotional well-being and even your financial status!

As well, her web site is loaded with information regarding stress relief, self-hypnosis techniques, ancient esoteric texts, and even CD's that stimulate your body's own built-in higher intelligence to change your physical form, i.e. breast enlargement, growth in height, weight management, hair growth and more!

If you smoke, you must quit at least two weeks prior to your surgery. I recommend trying Dr. DiGiorgio's Stop Smoking CD or other non-medicinal methods, as you don't want to pollute your body prior to your surgery.

Even if you don't have surgery, you must quit smoking (assuming that you do smoke). Nothing will age your face and teeth, not to mention your internal organs, like smoking does. If you want to look your best and stay that way, you have got to quit smoking…NOW! I smoked for 11 years; from the time I was 12 years old until I was 23.

I quit when my father died…watching him rot away of cancer, still puffing on a Marlboro Light up until the hour he was too weak to raise his hand to his lips anymore was enough for me.

Please have enough love and respect for yourself and your family to do whatever you need to do to get that homicidal monkey off your back. Okay, I'll stop preaching now! ☺

…And Don't Forget to Bring Your Toothbrush! (Things to Bring for Your Cosmetic Surgery Trip to the Dominican Republic)

Packing for any vacation is a real chore and an exercise in resourcefulness to say the least! In the case of a plastic surgery vacation, it takes some real foresight and preparedness to make sure you have the supplies you need to make your recovery as smooth and comfortable as possible.

Some of the things you absolutely should bring with you include: Clothing appropriate to the surgery you will be having, i.e. caftans or loose fitting nightgowns and casual dresses if you are having tummy tuck, thigh lift, liposuction, breast reduction or augmentation.

Also, if you have any work done involving your breasts or arms, you must take into consideration that you will not be able to raise your arms easily, if at all!

You may need to get creative in your style of dress…maybe something sleeveless and roomy that buttons all the way up the front. Don't worry what you look like; your main concern is comfort and proper healing. You must not jeopardize your long-term results over short-term vanity.

Take it from me, I had absolutely no idea what to bring with me when I had my arm lift, and I went through a lot of unnecessary pain and stretching of my suture lines because I brought clothes that were difficult to put on and take off. My scars are now quite wider than I had hoped they would be because of this and the fact that I didn't keep my compression garment on the way I should have. Please! Learn from my mistakes!

Just buying clothes that are a few sizes too big is not good enough! You really have to think through the movements that you make taking the clothes off and putting them on.

Buy stretchy, lightweight knits as opposed to tight-weave cottons that do not give when you move. You can sometimes find some great outfits in this category at Blair.com

Oh! I almost forgot something very, very important…do yourself a BIG favor and only bring slip on shoes! You will not want to be bending over to try and tie or buckle shoes or sandals! And most likely, after all the help you will be asking for from others, you'll be happy to be able to put your shoes on all by yourself.

You also may want to have a box or two of super-absorbent maxi-pads if you have liposuction, arm lift or thigh lift. I really wished I had a box when I had my arm lift and back liposculpture, because the drainage was horrendous! I soaked towel after towel, and had a really difficult time just trying to keep dry. It was pretty gross, but I just couldn't bring myself to send my husband out for a box of Kotex!

I would have liked to have had some of those absorbent bed liners (the kind with the white cotton top and the blue plastic backing). I was sharing a bed in the hotel with my husband and was constantly paranoid that his side of the bed was going to get soaked…unneeded stress to be sure!

My doctor gave me quite a lot of gauze bandages, but to be on the safe side you should bring plenty of your own, as well as cotton surgical dressing, surgical tape, and your own ACE bandages. You may not need it all, but you will feel better and more comfortable knowing you are well prepared! Baby wipes, antibiotic ointment, good moisturizing lotion, hydrogen peroxide and Q-tips are all good to have on hand. Also, bring an ample supply of Tylenol and Advil. You're going to need it!

One of my recent discoveries that has absolutely changed my life is a microdermabrasion cloth. This thing is an absolute MIRACLE! I had such problems with my skin…breakouts, dry patches, and scabs. Yick, it was just horrible. I had been seeing this microdermabrasion cloth advertised on eBay a lot and I said to myself, "That's got to be a load of crap." How could a cloth do all the things they claimed…getting rid of acne, scars, wrinkles, giant pores? This is one product that really WORKS!

I broke down and bought one and I saw an amazing difference in my skin after the very first use. My bumps went away, my scars healed, the red spots, blackheads, scabs, pits (God, I sound disgusting! But my skin was bad, man!)…They are all gone. I am living my dream of not having to wear foundation! Yeah! My skin looks better than it did in high school.

This towel literally sucks the dirt out of your pores! You think you're getting your face clean when you wash with soap, but you're not! The soap just builds up and clogs your pores, trapping the oil and bacteria in there. Well, I literally have not used soap in a week and I am cleaner than ever. My skin just glows now!

So I was thinking, this is an absolute MUST HAVE ITEM for after your surgery because it gets you so clean. It just has to be a little damp with water and you can use it all over your body (except those delicate areas, of course) and it gets you cleaner than anything else possibly could!

One of the yuckiest parts of surgery is not feeling clean for so many days/weeks after surgery when you can't take a bath. But this towel will be the remedy for that! I promise! It is great.

Now, you can buy most of all the above stuff here…probably quite a bit cheaper, too! But most people are not going to want to shuffle around a city they are unfamiliar with to get all of this stuff when they are about to undergo surgery. Your mind will be elsewhere, so to speak.

Having said all that, I must stress that you should travel as lightly as possible! You do not want to have to worry about lugging a giant, heavy suitcase around with you as you trudge through the airport. It will cause you great stress and agony on the flight home, which you do not need.

A nightgown or two and a change of clothes to wear for your return home should be plenty. You are going to spend most of your time in bed recovering, so don't worry about making any fashion statements.

Keep your toiletries as light as possible, too. Do yourself a favor and limit your luggage to a carry on. You'll be glad you did.

Use Your (Recovery) Time Wisely

Regardless of which type of surgery you are going to undergo, you most likely are going to have a lot of empty hours on your hands (the likes of which you are probably not accustomed to). Instead of driving yourself nuts wanting to "get up and do something", change your attitude and you can get a lot more out of the entire experience.

Take this time for yourself…for your own mental and emotional "retreat". Bring books about subjects you've always wanted to learn a little more about but never carved out the time for. Indulge yourself in meditation CD's and personal growth training. Bring a notebook and do some personal journaling…either about the experience you are going through or about deep personal issues you have buried in your mind that are in need of excavation.

Another great idea is to bring your favorite audio books. You'll have times when you don't even want to have your eyes open, but you will want some mental stimulation. Audiobooks are great!

By the way, if you are into reading a lot on your computer check out **ReadPlease.com,** where you can download a little program that you can copy and paste documents and web site text and the software will read it to you out loud! And it's free!

You should definitely check it out. They offer a version of the program that will even record the text in an MP3 format so you can record books or online information and burn it on a CD…in essence make your own audio books! I use mine every day and I get so much more done. It's amazing.

Make this trip about YOU…physically, mentally, emotionally and spiritually. You are so much more than just a body that needs "repair". The world is so screwed up right now, and we have all had to work so much harder than ever just to stay afloat and keep our kids and spouses healthy and happy, you owe it to yourself to be a "diva" for a change!

Uncover your inner artist. My all-time favorite book on this process is **"The Artist's Way"**, by Julia Cameron. That book helped me write this one!

Give yourself a chance to daydream. Bring a little sketchbook and do some doodling.

Figure out what may not be working in your life and brainstorm on ways to improve it! The guru on this subject is Tony Robbins. I have used his tapes since 1996, and I have to tell you he really helped me turn things around! I don't think I would ever have had the courage to go through all of this if it hadn't been for his techniques. Every once in a while I go back to those tapes when I need a "power boost"!

We are all sweet, delicate creatures that need nurturing…but unless you make that your own responsibility, you're likely not going to get what you need. I guess what I'm trying to share with you, is that from experience I have found that being dissatisfied with your physical body occurs in direct correlation with being dissatisfied with something else. Fixing one does not automatically fix the other.

I recently discovered the work of the late Dr. Maxwell Maltz, one of the pioneers of plastic surgery in the United States. Following the progress of his patients post-plastic surgery, Dr. Maltz was intrigued by the way some patients would completely change in personality following the improvement of their physical appearance. Phobias and inhibitions would sometimes fade completely and the patients would begin life anew with confidence and optimism they never possessed prior to surgery.

However, Dr. Maltz also noted that some of his patients not only didn't gain confidence following their successful surgeries, but actually couldn't *see* any difference in their appearances no matter how outwardly dramatic the change was! Their self-concept and self-image was stuck in the same place it had been prior to surgery. It would take years of psychotherapy to help some of these patients.

Dr. Maltz went on to write the classic self-improvement book **"Psychocybernetics"**. Although the title is a little intimidating, the text is easy to read and quite eye-opening. It really hit home with me. The basic idea is that only by mentally changing one's self-image can one achieve anything that has been "programmed out" of your realm of possibilities.
Having studied self-help and self-improvement doctrines for over 10 years now, I know this is the main underlying theme through them all.

But hearing these ideas coming from a plastic surgeon himself gave it all more depth for me. It has taken a good, long time for me to start to see myself the way others see me. I still feel slightly self-conscious about my body. The little fat girl still whispers in the back of my mind occasionally. But I stay dedicated to working through my past negative "programming" with self-hypnosis and subliminal recordings nightly and I believe that is why my life has improved as much as it has and I am finally attracting the kinds of opportunities that have been coming my way recently. Anything you want, you can have…but you have to *allow* yourself to receive it!

If you use your recovery time to its fullest, the rewards will far more profound than just getting a flat tummy or a younger face!

I believe so strongly in the power of the human mind…the brain is just like a computer. And as every computer geek likes to preach, "Garbage in – Garbage out"! Because of my passion for personal growth and mind management, I have invested in a huge library of self-help books, tapes, CD's, DVD's and videotapes that I am sure have saved my life from time to time.

Devoting so much time and effort to healing my emotional pain and redirecting my consciousness in a positive way has made such a difference in my life, I feel very compelled to help others conquer their fears and self-doubts so they can experience life in a rich and rewarding way.

Of course, I don't force these ideas on anyone, but I am very supportive of those who really want to learn techniques for making life as enjoyable and happy as possible!

A Little Advice on "After-Care"

To help your wounds heal into the smallest, lightest scar possible, try lightly coating them with olive oil daily (of course, you need to wait until they are completely healed…at least 3 weeks post-operatively). A good over-the-counter remedy for scar reduction is Mederma.

As your wounds heal to the point when you can cover them with make-up, the best cover-up is **Dermablend**. They have colors to match almost every skin type, and the coverage is really, really good.

One thing you may not be aware of…liposuction does not always improve the look of cellulite, and can even make the appearance of thigh dimples more pronounced!

Make sure that you wear your compression garment as instructed by your doctor. Even when you're able to finally take it off, you should continue to wear support pantyhose.

I found that a hand-held ultrasonic massager is indispensable in your recovery period following liposuction. Following my last lipo, the doc told me it was important for me to start getting massages…*ultrasonic* massages!

I thought I knew a lot about such things, but I really had never heard much about ultrasonic massage. I was in a car accident about 7 years ago and the physical therapist I had to see used it on me, but I didn't pay much mind to it.

I panicked a little when I contemplated having to go to a salon every day for these special treatments. You know how I hate to spend too much money! I decided to do a little investigating and see if it was possible for me to get my own ultrasonic massager at a price that would save me some money in the long run.

As I searched the Internet, I found some units cost as much as $10,000.00!! Yipes! I thought then that I was going to be shelling out for my daily sessions. Always the optimist, I continued my Internet search. I found some units at $675.00, $390.00, and $275.00. I was getting encouraged now...but I had to keep looking for one that was even lower in price.

I took a chance and searched my favorite web site, EBAY! Wouldn't you know it?? There was an ultrasonic massager, the same model as the one I found elsewhere for over $300.00. How much was it on EBay, you ask? Only $55.00! EBay has saved me again! I was still a little skeptical, but I took the chance and bought it.

After only two treatments, I saw a major difference in myself. What kind of difference? Well, it is common following liposuction to have some areas of unevenness, dimpling and swelling. I had this big time at the base of my back, just above my butt.

My ultrasonic massager made my back so much smoother! It was almost unbelievable! I was so glad that I bought that thing...I couldn't stand the thought of having to keep an appointment every day, get naked in front of some stranger, and pay between $5 and $10 a session (cheap here in the DR; in the US you can pay upwards of $80 per session from what I've read)!

Just like every time I buy something, I found it even less expensive today! I found it for just over $45.00. On the internet, go to the web site **http://www.apexdistributiongroup.com**. This is the same company I bought mine from off of EBay.

It turns out that the ultrasonic massager is marketed as a treatment to reduce fat by deep heat vaporization, as well as providing a deep massage and diminishing facial wrinkles and acne! I must attest, I believe it is getting rid of the little blurb of double chin I have as well as toning up my face!

I highly recommend ultrasonic massage. I have happily made it part of my daily routine. You must use it with a conductive gel (which I also found on EBay for $15.00 for a big 5-liter bottle). It is recommended that you only use it for a total of 15 minutes at one time.

One Last Word About Dominican Plastic Surgeons (the Inside Scoop)

I would like to reiterate one final point...I was absolutely astounded by the quality of care that I received and the level of compassion and concern that I was treated with in the Dominican Republic. All of the Dominican plastic surgeons that I have met and dealt with both throughout my surgeries and in researching and writing this book really impressed me with their level of professionalism and ethical conduct.

When approached regarding being included in this book, none of them were particularly eager to be singled out. Each felt that any form of "advertising" (which they deemed this to be) is unethical for any professional...doctor, lawyer, etc.

Even though I tried my best to explain to them that I was writing the book with no bias toward any particular surgeon and not as any kind of service to them, just as a personal account and an informative guide for those interested in finding high quality cosmetic surgery in the Dominican Republic, they still kept me and my little project ever-so pleasantly at arms length.

Evidently, each of them is proud of the fact that he (or she, as the case may be) has built a healthy practice and an esteemed reputation solely from producing excellent results and happy patients. This is even more reason to be reassured by their level of quality and integrity (although it did make my job a little more challenging).

When I asked one surgeon if he could direct me to another few physicians whom he regarded to be especially good his reply was, "We're all good." I liked that.

And take no offense if a Dominican plastic surgeon seems a little hesitant to take you on at first...there is a sad situation out there in the world created by politicians and the media that is not doing you any good on a personal level.

Americans have developed a worldwide reputation as being coarse, nasty, malevolent and extremely eager to unjustly sue the pants off of everyone and anyone for totally fabricated reasons.

I believe the majority of Americans are sweet, compassionate and law-abiding people. Unfortunately, governmental policy and obnoxious criminals grab all the headlines and are giving the rest of us a bad name in the process. It's only too often we see stories on the New York news about people who have faked injuries or even caused their own injuries in effort to scam an insurance company, not caring whose hard-earned medical career and reputation is laid to waste in the process.

This is one of the major reasons that medical care of any kind is so outrageously costly in the US right now. The lawsuits have gotten out of control and in my opinion have done irreparable damage to the system and to the quality of work being performed by American doctors in general. And if you think all the pressure of the threat of million-dollar lawsuits doesn't or shouldn't affect the quality of a physician or surgeon's performance, I urge you to consider the following.

Have you ever driven for 12-14 hours or more without a moment's rest, through dangerous traffic and weather conditions, perhaps with kids screaming and fighting in the backseat? Do you remember the way you felt? The fear and anxiety that courses through your body, and the knowledge that one mistake could cost your family or some other innocent person or people on the road their very lives? And it would be your fault?

Now think of what it must be like to operate on that level, day after day…with hospital administrators constantly and unkindly reminding you that if you "screw up" even once it could cost some patient her life (or lessen the quality thereof), could cost you your career and everything you've worked for, as well as costing the hospital millions of dollars.

It was recently reported in the Journal of the American Medical Association that doctors and hospitals ranked in the top 5 leading causes of death in America!

In fact, last year or so well-known author Olivia Goldsmith, who wrote "The First Wives' Club", died during induction of anesthesia during her facelift operation at the Manhattan Eye, Ear and Throat Hospital. I mention this not to exploit the death of Ms. Goldsmith, but to drive home the point that paying a lot of money and/or having your cosmetic surgery in the United States does not guarantee safety or results.

So those who think that having surgery performed in America ensures a better outcome than having surgery performed in any other country of the world are sadly deluding themselves.

In fact, I have read on various plastic surgery message boards countless stories of people who had poor results and/or complications following their cosmetic surgery only to have their (American) doctor refuse to take their phone calls afterward!

American doctors have my most sincere sympathy for their plight…high malpractice insurance premiums, high cost of operating a medical office, etc. makes for higher prices to charge their patients. However, you don't have to play that game and put yourself and your family in thousands and thousands of dollars of debt so you can get the surgery you want and need. The word "American" does not necessarily mean "better" or "safer". The US media has conditioned us to believe that, but don't fall prey to their manipulation.

Besides the benefits of having great cosmetic surgery performed by talented Board Certified plastic surgeons for rock bottom prices, there lie even more glorious reasons to have your surgery in the Dominican Republic…anonymity, movie-star treatment and the option to spend your recovery period in a tropical paradise!

It is well know to many of the world's rich and famous that the people of the Dominican Republic are very unaffected by their celebrity status. In fact, ex-pres Bill Clinton brought the family here for Easter vacation, after having spent New Year's vacation here along with ex-pres. Jimmy Carter and his clan! Ex-American presidents are flocking to the DR for their R&R lately, as George Bush, Sr. made a visit to one of the country's most prestigious golf courses quite recently.

Michael Jackson and Lisa Marie Presley were married here. Mike Tyson was divorced here. Singer Shakira is said to be buying over 200 acres of beachfront property in the DR, as are Senator Hilary Clinton and her husband, former US pres. Bill. Some other notables such as Sean (Puffy, P Diddy, Puff Daddy, whatever he likes to be called) Combs and Liz Taylor also visited last year, although I don't think they were together...

My point is not to name drop (as much as I do enjoy that), but to emphasize the fact that you can come to the Dominican Republic and enjoy your privacy, have your cosmetic surgery here and nobody back home even needs to know about it. Stay long enough for your bruising and swelling to diminish and no one will be any the wiser. Your friends, family and co-workers will just think you had a fantastic vacation that "worked wonders for you".

If you choose to spend your recovery time at one of the country's all-inclusive beachfront resorts, you won't be able to lounge on the beach or belly-up to the pool bar, you can at least enjoy a gorgeous ocean view from your balcony, enjoy all-you-can-eat smorgasbords (if you don't mind turning a few heads) and when you feel up to it you can get out for some short scenic walks in the shade (if your doctor approves) and a little socializing.

Be advised, however, that you will most likely be in for at least a 40 minute drive to reach the nearest all-inclusive beachfront resort if you have your surgery done in Santo Domingo or Santiago (which may be uncomfortable if you try it too soon after certain surgical procedures). It would be best to consult with your surgeon prior to making such plans.

There are many casinos, a fantastic zoo and aquarium, underground caves, baseball games, cultural centers, world-class shopping, and tropical sight-seeing trips that you can take advantage of if you are feeling frisky before your surgery…but you probably won't be up to any of that post-op.

For major procedures or a combination of a few procedures, I must tell you that you most likely will feel like staying cozily in your bed for the majority of your stay. However, it is good to know that if you bring friends or family they will have plenty to see and do while you are recovering from your surgery!

Globalization and *You*

Shortly after I moved to the Dominican Republic, I watched a speech being given by former US president Bill Clinton as he addressed the British Parliament regarding the concept of "Globalization". He urged the crowd to embrace and encourage more open trade agreements and generally higher tolerance and increased friendliness with all other nations of the world. The advent of the internet has indeed shrunk the world even smaller than the advent of the airplane did 100 years ago. We're now able to buy items directly from China, Pakistan or India with a few clicks of a mouse. Few people have stopped to consider the implications on their own lives.

Some of us are leary and fearful of anything "foreign". Again, this is part of our programming. It doesn't help that our government has not garnered a very friendly reputation in the rest of the world. Luckily, though, most fairly developed nations do not hold it against us, the citizens of the United States. America has made great contributions to the quality of life around the world and for the most part we are still highly regarded for such.

I have to admit, I have spent considerable time researching the political movement of "Globalization". The conspiracy theories on the subject are quite negative, and for the first couple of years that I studied it all, I was getting scared. Plots for world domination and plans for "population control" are foreboding. To be honest, it was getting me paranoid and depressed.

Now, I of course don't know whether the intentions of the Globalization movement are sinister and evil or meant to ultimately promote world peace. One thing I do believe is that it can be a very good thing if we as average citizens of the world become more tolerant of our differences and stay focused on mutually beneficial dealings with each other. Fear and hatred are just about played out and the closer we get to peace, love and understanding the better off we will all be.

At the forefront of the Globalization movement is the trend of medical tourism. Growing in strength yearly, medical tourism is now big business as more and more average people from "overdeveloped countries" find themselves literally forced to fly to other countries to receive the medical care that has priced them out of the United States, Great Britain, etc. Countries including India, Thailand, the Dominican Republic, Mexico, Brazil, Indonesia, Venezuela, Costa Rica, Panama, Turkey, South Africa and others are becoming destinations for those who are not willing to lose their homes or go deeply in debt for the rest of their lives in order to have major or minor surgeries.

Already a multi-billion dollar industry, medical tourism is growing by roughly 30% each year and showing no signs of slowing. Traveling patients are finding that their journeys save them many thousands of dollars and they are receiving excellent medical and surgical care. Competition is now global for everything, including hip replacements and nose jobs. The playing field is being leveled. In fact, many of the doctors and surgeons who are treating traveling patients are doctors who were trained in American universities and hospitals and have now returned to their home countries to practice medicine.

We are in the midst of sweeping changes throughout the world. There is sure to be backlash, mainly from the medical establishments of the countries that are losing patients to medical tourism. One of the biggest drawbacks of seeking any kind of medical or surgical care outside one's country of origin is the lack of long-term follow-up care when you arrive back home. Some jilted US physicians are refusing to treat patients who have had surgery elsewhere. This, of course, is contrary to the basic medical ethics that we all have come to expect from our family doctors.

As an example of the gross patient neglect that is occurring, a patient who needed follow-up care in America after having had plastic surgery in Mexico was told by a local doctor that he would not treat her and she should "go to a veterinarian"! How horrible! These are these are the "caring" professionals that we are supposed to be mortgaging our houses to pay? It is behavior like that which is encouraging, not dissuading, people to seek medical, surgical and dental care in countries where patients are treated with respect.

So, in spite of the media sensationalism and negative stories being spread around, people with the intelligence and financial savvy to see through the fear-mongering are embracing new options and saving themselves and their families from poverty-inducing overpriced health services at home.

Dominican Republic Travel FAQ's

Where is the Dominican Republic, and What is it Like?

The Dominican Republic is in the Caribbean. It is located on the island of Hispañola and covers an area of about the size and shape of New York State. The only other country on the island is Haiti, which is our neighbor to the west. However, the Dominican Republic is a lush tropical paradise, rich in natural resources as opposed to Haiti, which is mostly desert and arid, unpalatable land. The two countries are like night and day, and the Dominican Republic does not have as much poverty or political upheaval as Haiti.

Is Spanish the Only Language Spoken in DR?

The DR (as commonly referred to by people in the States) is mainly Spanish speaking, but most people who work in the travel and tourism industry speak several languages including English, German, French and Italian! Also, many professionals (doctors, lawyers, etc.) speak English and French as well as Spanish.

Who Goes There For Vacation?

The Dominican Republic is actually experiencing a huge rise in popularity with American travelers, because the exchange rate is facilitating very, very inexpensive luxury vacations. In fact, the tourism industry has just announced that the DR is the most popular tourist destination in the Caribbean, playing host to 3.6 million tourists in 2005, mostly from America but also from Canada, England and Europe! The DR has been considered the "Best Kept Secret of the Caribbean", since most of the tourists and investors here have been of European origin for many years.

What is the Government Like?

The government is democratic. The judicial system is based on the French law system. The people and government are very, very friendly and respectful towards tourists. As an American, Canadian, Brit or other foreign traveler, you will find yourself treated like a 'special guest' almost certainly!

How Far Away is it and What Airlines Can I Use to Get There?

The DR is one of the northernmost Caribbean countries, with only Cuba being closer to the US. You can fly here from New York in about 3 hours and 15 minutes, or from Miami in about 2 and ½ hours. American Airlines is the major carrier, and flies many flights in and out every day.

Most recently, economical airline JetBlue has begun twice-daily flights between New York's JFK airport and both Santiago, which is about an hour and a half drive from Santo Domingo. Current fares are very low starting at $99.00 each way! I am a big fan of JetBlue, as the planes are brand new, each seat has a TV, there's plenty of legroom, and the staff is friendly. Oh, and they are almost always on time!

What City Should I Fly Into if I'm Going for Plastic Surgery?

Most of the plastic surgery is performed in either the country's capital, Santo Domingo in the south or the second largest city, Santiago which is towards the north. You would fly into Las Americas Airport (Airport Code SDQ) if having surgery in Santo Domingo, and the Santiago Airport (Airport Code STI) if having surgery in Santiago.

How Much Will It Cost to Fly to the DR?

The travel industry is crazy…I have seen plane tickets for as low as $250.00 from Tampa to Santo Domingo. I have also seen tickets as high as $1,600.00 for the same route! My best suggestion is to plan ahead and do plenty of research, including using online sources as well as your local travel agent. Prices are unpredictable in the travel industry and you never know where the best deal is going to come from!

How Much Will it Cost for Ground Transportation, Like from the Airport to the Hotel?

Average taxi rates for the trip from the Las Americas Airport to the largest hotels of Santo Domingo are about $25.00-$35.00 USD by taxi one-way. Various destinations in Santo Domingo (i.e. between your hotel and plastic surgery clinic) should cost no more than $2.50. I suggest you check out **http://www.dominicantaxi.com** to set up your ground transportation before you arrive. That will take lots of worry out of your trip!

How Much Will a Hotel Cost for Two Weeks in Santo Domingo?

Hotel rates vary quite dramatically. While you can find lower class rooms in small hotels for only $55.00 a night, Santo Domingo has quite a few exquisite 5-star hotels that can cost upwards of $200.00 or more per night, per person (even more for special suites). It is all a matter of your personal standards.

Personally, I feel it is worth spending a little extra to make sure that your stay is as luxurious as you will allow yourself to afford. You are going to need peace and pleasant surroundings to heal in the optimal time frame. Risking your peace of mind to save a couple of hundred dollars is not worth it in my book. You need to look for something ultra-clean, ultra-comfortable, and with a helpful, professional staff that is willing to go the extra yard for you.

For example, when I stayed at a hotel (the Hotel Hispañola) for my second surgery, breakfast was included with the price of the room. The breakfast buffet was awesome, with loads of fresh locally grown tropical fruit in every variety you can imagine as well as other local morning delicacies and pastries.

My husband, son and mother would go down to breakfast every morning and instead of making me wait for them to come back with a tray of food, my husband arranged (with the help of a wisely spent $3.00 tip) to have one of the waiters bring me a tray of goodies every morning. I really enjoyed that! With most surgeries, you're not even able to wash your hair or take a bath for a week at least…so the last thing you are going to want to do is go display your funky self in the buffet line.

If you have the self-discipline to stay out of the sun, there are several beautiful all-inclusive beach resorts about 45 minutes away from Santo Domingo. The hotel chain Barcelo has 3 resorts which range from small and quiet to large and luxurious. Prices include all meals and drinks which is a real plus, and if you bring your family they can go out and have a fun-filled Caribbean beach vacation while you are in bed healing. Prices range from $75.00 per person per night up to around $200.00 per night.

Another option that several of my readers have told me about is Casa De Huespedes, the private home of Ms. Angela Valentin. I have had the pleasure of meeting Ms. Valentin and she seems like a lovely lady. Christie, the star of the Canadian documentary I mentioned earlier, stayed with Angela following her first surgery with Dr. Guerrero and she was very happy with the accommodations, meals, transportation and personal care that was provided for one all-inclusive price of $55.00 per night. Contact information for Casa De Huespedes can be found in the **Resources** section at the end of this book.

How Much Will My Meals Cost?

Again, there are very cheap options and very expensive options in the gastronomical delights of the DR. Room service in an expensive hotel could cost up to $20.00 per meal or so. But the average restaurant meal in a modest place will cost around $4.00 to $8.00 USD.

Will I Be Covered By Any Insurance?

Chances are you will not be covered by any medical insurance for cosmetic surgery. Whether you will be covered by your own health insurance is dependent upon your carrier, with whom you should consult prior to your departure regarding what incidents you may be covered for.

I have heard stories of patients who had plastic surgery in the Dominican Republic that was approved and paid for (or reimbursed) by their insurance companies.

A good source for the best rates for travel insurance can be found online by visiting the following URL on the internet:

http://insuremytrip.com/p/myquote?pid=5862

What Documents Do I Need to Travel to the DR?

Americans don't need visas or even a Passport to come to the DR, as you can fly on your birth certificate and driver's license as your only ID (however, I do recommend you have a passport as in these times you never know when they (the US) is going to abruptly pass a new travel-related law and you don't want to have to go through the red tape of getting a passport while you are here just so that you can get back home (of course, you may just fall in love with this place and want to stay forever like I did! LOL)

What is the International Calling Code to the Dominican Republic?

To call the Dominican Republic from the United States, there is no need to dial any international code. Just like calling a long distance phone number in America, dial 1-(809)-xxx-xxx. Currently there is only area code in the Dominican Republic, which is 809. To call from the United Kingdom, dial 00-809 + the number. To call from Canada, dial 011-809 + the number. To find other international dialing codes, visit **http://www.countrycallingcodes.com**.

Why Don't I Find More Information Online About Dominican Republic Plastic Surgeons?

The plastic surgeons here have no real need to advertise on the internet for new clients from other countries. They're proud of the fact that they are booked well with referrals from past patients, and they see advertising for patients as something that is unethical and unnecessary.

What Forms of Payment Do Dominican Plastic Surgeons Accept?

Most likely, the only form of payment that your Dominican Republic plastic surgeon will accept is cash in the form of Dominican Pesos. It is best to verify this ahead of time with your doctor before coming to the Dominican Republic.

I have found a service that delivers cash to recipients in the Dominican Republic via Paypal.com. The service called **Envios Boya**.

Please see their website **http://www.EnviosBoya.com** for further details regarding this service.

Buying Travelers' Checks ahead of time and exchanging them for cash in the Dominican Republic is another way to go.

Is There Anyway I Can Get Financing for My Plastic Surgery in the Dominican Republic?

I have recently discovered a financing company that is willing to finance surgery for patients who are using overseas surgeons! This is great news, as many of us can afford a fair monthly payment, but are not able to put together a chunk of cash for surgery (even if it is a much smaller chunk than that we'd fork over to a US plastic surgeon).

The company is called **Advanced Patient Financing**. They work with several large financing company to find just the right financing plan to work with your budget and credit history, and there is no pre-payment penalty, so if you should experience a windfall or want to use next year's tax return money to pay off your loan early they won't hold it against you and make you pay an early termination fee. Please see the Resources section at the back of the book for more information regarding **Advanced Patient Financing**.

Can I Consult With a DR Plastic Surgeon Without Leaving the United States?

There are several Dominican Plastic Surgeons who have web sites and more who have email addresses. I have listed as many of them as I could find towards the end of this book, along with the contact information for the surgeon, the address of the office/clinic and any other pertinent information I have been able to collect.

Several of these "internet savvy" surgeons are willing to do a virtual pre-consult via email, where you would send him or her photos of yourself via email and tell him/her what it is you would like to have done. The doctor can usually give you a pretty good idea of what can be done for you, when it can be done and how much it will cost.

I have heard of Dominican doctors who will consult with as many as 30 or more patients at once while just visiting in the States...sometimes at the request of former patients, they will visit with the former patients' friends and family members to give them a mini-consultation before the prospective patients head down to the DR!

This kind of situation usually occurs in US cities that have a high number of citizens of Dominican origin, like New York, Philadelphia, Rhode Island, Boston and Miami. Usually these are held at local beauty salons or private homes.

Tell Me About Dental Care in the DR!

I have also had the pleasure of getting superb dental care here in the Dominican Republic. In fact, I hadn't been to a dentist since I was 10 years old! My family could not afford regular dental care when I was a kid, and neither could I when I was an adult. Like many people, I thought of going to a dentist only out of agonizing pain (which I never had). I knew, however, that I must have a lot of cavities. I also had two ugly (not to mention DANGEROUS & POISONOUS) metal fillings that I got at that visit when I was 10.

When I moved to DR, I went to a dentist and to my dismay I found out that I needed fillings in almost every tooth in my head! Including my two front teeth! I was scared of the process and of how much it would cost. I also had ugly indentations at the top of my two front teeth that I was very self-conscious about, so I tried not to smile too much :(. In only 2 weeks of going to the dentist every few days (each visit lasting no longer than 20 minutes or so), I had a beautiful smile again!

They removed my ugly metal fillings and replaced them with nice white plastic, drilled and filled all of my teeth and fixed the deformed indentations of my front teeth! I only had 2 shots of Novocain throughout those 2 weeks and I had no pain. But here is the best part....the entire bill came to only $400.00!!! I couldn't believe it! I cannot imagine how much it would have cost me in the States, not to mention the fact that they would have dragged it out over a period of months or years.

I brought my mom with me when I got my arm lift and lipo, my second DR surgery trip. Her teeth were TERRIBLE! She was missing a few, had mismatched caps on several due to years of bad dental care in the US and had lots of problems. She needed a partial bridge, too. She had visited a dentist in Charlotte, North Carolina who told her it would take several years to fix her teeth and would cost at least $20,000.00! Here, the dentist did all the work she needed in only 5 days...total cost: $1,700.00! That was with a custom made bridge and all! Now she smiles all the time!

At the end of this book, you will find a listing of dentists, orthodontists and oral surgeons in the Dominican Republic who can provide affordable, high-quality dental care.

Other Money-Saving Surgery Options

Just because I found great surgery at great prices in the Dominican Republic doesn't mean that there aren't other options.

Below you will find the information I've gathered regarding some of the most popular worldwide destinations now becoming well known for their combination of affordability and safe surgery with good results.

Since my personal experience is limited to the Dominican Republic, I cannot comment on the abilities of the surgeons or the results you can expect. I have simply gathered lots of contact information and as many other details as I could to help you in your research.

South Africa

This is a great option for the truly adventurous plastic surgery seekers. South Africa has become a well-publicized destination for cosmetic surgery tourism in recent years.

At the end of this book, you will find some links to useful information and web sites I have discovered regarding plastic surgery resorts and facilities in the most southern portion of the Dark Continent.

Being advertised as a "Safari and Surgery Vacations", some facilities offer a real African safari prior to your surgery. Well, that *sounds* really cool to me because I love animals. My house has become home to a peacock, a baby iguana, two cockatiels, two obnoxious but lovable little parrots and two cats! However, combining surgery and safari is nothing I could handle emotionally.

Going under the knife stresses me out enough…add the possibility of being chased and/or eaten by lions is just too much excitement for my sensitive nervous system.

Of course, I'm sure if you're a little bit of a neurotic like me you can bow out of the safari part. Just make sure they take it off your bill at the end of your stay!

It was difficult for me to find much information regarding prices for individual surgical procedures in South Africa. However, I did scout up a magazine article that quoted a price of about $3,500.00 for breast augmentation surgery (which is just about $500.00 more than in the Dominican Republic).

Accommodations range between low budget and 5-star, prices from $414.00 to $866.00US per week.

The lowest priced airfare that I found was $1660.00 from JFK in New York City to Johannesburg for a 27-hour flight with a stop in London. You get there 2 days after you leave JFK.

This airfare was per person, economy class, priced one month in advance of the trip and staying for 2 weeks.

Costa Rica

It is true that Costa Rica has an internet presence as being a destination for Americans who want inexpensive cosmetic surgery.

The reason that Costa Rica is appealing to Americans more so than the Dominican Republic is two-fold...Costa Rica has been 'Americanized', i.e. for the past 25 years many American individuals and companies have invested in Costa Rica and have influenced the development of the country in that direction.

The Dominican Republic, on the other hand, has remained sovereign unto itself. By this I mean that it is not as overrun by American corporations (although that is changing fairly rapidly). For example, there are only two or three cities in the entire country where you will find a McDonald's.

I did some research and discovered that the prices in Costa Rica are an average of $1500-$2000 higher than in the Dominican Republic. This is based on a price list that I found on web site **http://www.zurqui.co.cr/crinfocus/plast/su-cos.html**.

However, the majority of the doctors here in the Dominican Republic do not base their prices on a "per procedure" rate. They will usually give you one price for ALL the procedures you want.

And the DR price also usually includes anesthesia, pre- and post-operative visits with the doctor, hospital stay, nursing, supplies, operating room costs, lab work, compression garments, etc.

I could not find any Costa Rica web site that said that they included all that. I did find one that says that they charge an extra $275.00 for any procedure requiring general anesthesia, an extra $90.00 for compression garment, and charge $1,900.00 for each area of liposuction.

So if I had it done in Costa Rica it would have cost me a minimum of $9,500.00, assuming that they would do all areas of my thighs for the same $1,900.00. Most American plastic surgeons consider inner thighs one area, outer thighs another area, etc.

If you are considering having your surgery in Costa Rica, I have found a web site of a surgical recovery retreat that looks very nice and has very reasonable prices.

The best airfare that I found was $503.00 JFK to San Jose stop in Panama for a 7-hour trip.

The price was based on a per person rate, economy class, priced one month in advance of the trip and staying for 2 weeks.

One of my readers, a very sweet and lovely former fashion model from California named EschaRose, sent me an email detailing her fantastic experience having several cosmetic surgery procedures in Costa Rica performed by her hero, Dr. Arnoldo Fournier. She is so thrilled with her results, as well as every other aspect of her trip, she encouraged me to share the following letter with you to pay homage to an excellent surgeon as well as help those looking for information regarding plastic surgery in Costa Rica. She wrote:

I OPENED WEB SITE OF DR. ARNOLDO FORNIER AND HIS PHOTO AND THE WORDS UNDER THE PHOTO AND HIS FACE CONNECTED ME TO HIM. WE CALLED AND IMMEDIATELY BEGAN LAUGHING AND TALKING OF MUSIC AND I WAS HOOKED. HE ASKED WHAT I NEEDED. I REMARKED, A FACE LIFT, UPPER AND LOWER EYES, TOTAL LIPO, AND TUMMY TUCK. HE SAID CAN YOU AFFORD 6,000--I WAS SMILING SO BIG--AND I ADDED I WOULD LIKE MY FACELIFT TO REFLECT BEAUTIFUL LIPS--HE SAID I WILL MAKE YOUR LIPS PERFECT AND LET´S SETTLE FOR 5,000!!! I BEGAN TO CRY. HE SAID COME NEXT WEEK AND YOU WILL BE MY QUEEN. I AM SERIOUS.

SO I ARRIVE THE 5TH, SANTA RITA HOSPITAL HAD NO PATIENTS. I WAS THE ONLY ONE. MADE UP MY ROOM AND THE PARTY BEGAN. NOT UNTIL 7 PM DID I SEE DR. FOURNIER--AND FOR THE REST OF MY LIFE I WILL SEND GIFTS--HONOR HIM AND SEND EVERYONE TO HIM. 5 HOUR SURGERY--EVERYTHING AT ONCE---NO PAIN--NONE--AND INCLUDED HAIR GRAFTS AND DERMADRASION ON LIPS THEN DERMALIFE INTO THE LIPS. I WAS DOWNSTAIRS ON THE EVENING OF THE 1ST NIGHT.

ON TUESDAY EARLY--I LEFT FOR MARTA QURIOS HOME---A
PEACEFUL HOME OF ELEGANCE AND THE TIME OF MY
LIFE. SHE AND I WILL ALWAYS REMAIN FRIENDS. I SAW
THE DR. EVERY OTHER DAY. MY WAIST IS 4 INCHES
SMALLER. MY FACE, EXACTLY AS THE PHOTO I E-MAILED
YOU MY LIPS ARE FOR A REVLON COMMERCIAL, AND I'M
SHRINKING AS WE SPEAK. THE HAIR TAKES 3 MONTHS.
BUT----JOANN-------I WENT TO CHE TICA (88 ACRES) RANCH TO
A RECOVERY HOME,(AN INVITE FOR LUNCH) AT 100 PER
DAY JUST BECAUSE THESE FOLKS LIVED NEXT DOOR TO
ME YEARS AGO--IT WAS HUGE BUT I PREFER TO HAVE A
WARM HOME WITH TWO FABULOUS KIDS AND OTHER
PATIENTS NEXT DOOR. MARTA'S WAS 50.00 PER DAY. SO
WHY DO I RAMBLE ON? DR. FOURNIER OFTEN KEPT ME
FOR I HOUR JUST TO TALK. HE SAID FINALLY------I HAVE
YOUR PHOTO AND I'M GOING TO RECOVER YOUR 30 YEAR
OLD FACE...HE DID.
 MY EXPERIENCE OF THIS COUNTRY WAS WONDERFUL.
THE SURGERY ROOM FOR 5-6 HOURS, AND 1 HALF DAYS
STAY WAS 1,400-----YOU WERE CORRECT. CHEAP AND
PERFECT. BUT, IF GOD EVER DESIGNED A MAN TO TAKE
CARE OF HIS PATIENTS IT IS DR. ARNOLDO. COME SEE
HIM. I WORKED OUT TODAY I HOUR. I'M SO HAPPY I COULD
BURST. WENT OUT AND BOUGHT JEWELRY. SO-------HOW
ARE YOU AND TELL ME EVERYTHING YOU ARE DOING.
WE WILL TALK AGAIN VERY SOON. THANKS TO YOU,

*DEAR, I MADE MY DREAM COME TRUE WITH THE FINEST
PLASTIC SURGEON LIFE COULD OFFER.
MANY HUGS,
 ESCHAROSE*

Mexico

Now, you can save yourself some money by going to Mexico for plastic surgery. My husband's cousin (the same one who first had liposuction in the Dominican Republic), has been living in Mexico for the past several years and she has had some work done by a couple of different plastic surgeons there.

What's the scoop? Okay…she says that the doctors she has met have been good, the prices were just a little higher than in the Dominican Republic, but they don't "suck enough" (i.e. they don't get as much fat out when they do liposuction).

All you have to do is watch a Spanish soap opera (novella) and you will see how incredibly beautiful all the women are. It's not just good genes…although that is a big part of it!

Of course there are an amazing number of naturally beautiful women of Spanish lineage.

But when you see a woman on TV that looks like she's 29 years old and find out that she's been acting on the same soap opera (novella) for 35 years, you figure it out. There are some amazing plastic surgeons in the

Spanish-speaking world and their portfolios are available on any Spanish language TV channel.

However, I found online that in Mexico the cost of tumescent liposuction (which doesn't get as much fat out as ultrasonic liposuction) is $2,000.00. The source I found did not say if this was per area or all-over. For me, that ends the discussion right there. Costs more, suck less. I'll take DR.

Tee Hee…just kidding!

If you live close to Mexico (i.e. California or Southwest US), it may be worth it for you to go South of the Border as there are probably travel savings involved, as well as shorter trips. That would be your call.

I have an extensive list of Mexican Board Certified plastic surgeons at the end of this book to help in that regard.

The lowest price I found for airfare was $463.00 JFK to Mexico City with a stop in Detroit, for a total trip time 7 hours and 30 minutes.

Again, that price is per person, economy class, priced one month in advance of the trip and staying for 2 weeks.

Thailand

Originally contributed to my online newsletter, **"Beautiful on a Budget"** by one of my readers, Captain Bud Zumwalt, I have chosen to add the following article in its entirety. At the end of this book is a listing of various plastic surgeons and plastic surgery clinics in Thailand.

"I am 54 but look 35 thanks to quality, but cheap surgery in Bangkok, Thailand. Within recent months, I underwent full-face lift, eyelid bags removal, lip injections, new chin, hair transplantation, and two nose jobs. Not that I looked all that bad before, but I was getting older looking.

Some of us made the discovery a long time ago that US Surgeons are expensive, totally off the wall cost wise, and in many cases not that competent or skilled. Our US Hospitals stink, compared to Bangkok, Thailand and the kind of care I got while there was outstanding!
Thai people not only go out of their way to help you, but also are always smiling!

I just got an excellent nose job (with all costs included) for $2500, and chin implant for $1000. I know that butt augmentation is $2500, breast augmentation $2200 with 500 CC implants included, eye lid upper and lower $350 each eye, etc. etc., lipo is $1000.

Again, these prices are ALL-INCLUSIVE, meaning you don't pay extra for Anesthesiology, Operating Room, ancillary personnel, medications, supplies, and what-not like they charge you in the US.
A round trip ticket is $840, hotel is $12 daily, steak dinner is $3.50. I might add that the airline flight to Bangkok is daily on some US Airlines, but it is a 30-hour trip.

The prices for various surgeries are usually listed on the web sites, so you know before leaving. Some prices are in USD others in Thai Bath currency, with an exchange of about 41 Bath equaling one US dollar. The hospitals are very advanced and the care is far superior to that which you receive in the USA. All operations include everything medically, plus many of the clinics take care of taxis, food, and the doctors even come to the hotel with the health care people to change your bandages! If they need to see you at the clinic, they send someone to pick you up with free transportation.

Only the clinics offer the escort English speaking Thai lady for your assistance. The hospitals do not do all that, but you are more assured of a quality job.

One doctor, after my two-week recovery period, hired a tour guide and gave me a free tour of Bangkok…including a free lunch! Many of the doctors will arrange to have someone to take you shopping as well. Make sure you get good references from anyone running a clinic before using one.

I do recommend both Dr. Suporn, who runs a reputable clinic, and Dr. Preechra, who runs his clinic at the Nursing Home Hospital.

Bangkok Hospital is a very good private hospital with an International Department for Westerners. Yan Hee is another one that I recommend. Plastic surgery is usually done at one of the well-equipped and very modern hospitals.

There is no need for any appointment.

Surgery is usually performed the afternoon following your first visit with the doctor. You talk over price in the morning and then they perform the surgery that same day! No delays! They even work weekends.

If one does a search of Plastic Surgery Thailand, many clinics, hospitals and other web sites will appear. Most all Thai doctors have web sites and email, so it is very easy to communicate with them from a far distance.

Also and perhaps most importantly, most Thai doctors speak English. All professionals in the country speak good English, as well many RNs and even lower level staff can speak with you.

Some doctors answer their own email, while others have consultants who answer the email for them, usually within 12 hours of receiving it.

Most Plastic Surgeons in Thailand are Board Certified.

Dental work is superior to ours and costs nothing but pennies in comparison. Dental work is done on a walk in basis, minus any need for appointment, usually within one half hour. I had 12 cavities done in two days, with a female dentist who bowed to me after she finished!

Thailand is known as the sex change Capital of the World, but they as well are highly skilled in other body parts. Since I am a male and wanted facial work I found out Thailand doctors were best suited to work on the male face, since most transgenders are males changing appearance to females.

However, these doctors have about a 50 percent generic female following, many ladies from America and European women, so don't think they only work on males.

The majority of photos on their sites are females. Straight males who are not transsexuals (who as well want to look their best) understand that these doctors know best how to make a male look good.

Many of the doctors were trained here in the states, but their prices reflect the Thai economy. The per-capita average personal income of a Thai is approximately $1,950.00/year, what most American's make in two or three weeks.

Unfortunately, many American's have no basic health care, only the rich and famous among us can afford American prices for Plastic Surgery here, and many Americans have to go without even basic dental care needs.

Like our manufacturing has gone overseas, including my own manufacturing job which I lost many years ago to that trend, we too must go abroad for quality dental work and plastic surgery that is affordable. 'Made in America' no longer applies to manufactured goods or your new face or body....LOL"

Venezuela

Looking for bigger butt cheeks? It seems that the Caribbean International Plastic Surgery Centre on Margarita Island in Venezuela is seeking to carve out place of prominence in the buttock augmentation field (pun intended).

I have no first hand, second hand or third hand info on the surgeries or facilities of this particular clinic other than from their own web site. However, I can tell you that their web site is very informative about the various methods of buttock augmentation. No costs are provided on the site.

Recently, I became acquainted with a service called Surgical Services International (SSI), and I'm quite impressed with the services they offer as well as the caring, friendly nature of the proprietors, Robert Strong and Tonya Peterson.

Also based on Margarita Island, Robert and Tonya tailor their service to the needs of each patient. They arrange for airport transfer, accommodations and meals at one of several beautiful beach resorts, as well as scheduling your surgery with the best surgeon for your particular surgery. They do not work for any particular clinic or doctor. They work for the patient. And they tell me they have done extensive research to find the best surgeons with the best prices. They even provide their patients with a cell phone programmed with speed dial for quick access to themselves and the doctors/clinics whom will perform your surgery.

They have a fantastic web site that I recommend you visit, **http://www.surgicalservicesinternational.com** and if you talk to Robert or Tonya, tell them JoAnn from the Dominican Republic referred you!

What about airfare, you ask? Best price I found was $525 JFK to Caracas stop in Miami with 9 hour 24 minute flight time.

Same as with the other flight criteria… per person, economy class, priced one month in advance of the trip and staying for 2 weeks.

Head for the Hills…But *Not* Beverly Hills!

If you are absolutely deathly afraid of the thought of going outside the United States for surgery, first stop being such a fraidy cat! Get out and see the world a little for Pete's sake! Just kidding.

If you live in a large city, i.e. New York, Miami, L.A., Chicago, Dallas, etc., you've got a whole lot of things working against you in regards to finding affordable plastic surgery.

First off…big city surgeons have to pay big city rents for posh big city offices, not to mention having to pay higher salaries to their employees who also have to pay big city rents.

Not only that, but in the big city (where the big bucks are made), plastic surgeons attract people who can afford to pay high prices for their surgery without batting a (droopy) eyelid. This drives the prices up, up, up!

That's why that disgusting troll-man dermatologist/pseudo-surgeon I went to see on the Upper West Side of Manhattan six years ago could afford to charge a $6,000.00 fee for doing next to nothing. I swear, I looked at his before and after portfolio and had to ask which was the "before" and which was the "after"! He's probably charging $12,000.00 now for sucking (he sucked alright…and I'm not talking about liposuction!)

I just get so mad when I think about how that idiot humiliated me and told me for 6 grand he could only suck out 2-4 lbs. of fat from my thighs and that he could never make me a "skinny minnie"…and Dr. Gonzales just made me 25 lbs. lighter in one session and only charged me $1,500.00 for everything! And treated me with respect and dignity! But I digress…

Back to the subject of saving money without leaving the States, you can save a substantial amount if you visit a small town plastic surgeon.

I'm not talking about trying to find a plastic surgeon in the Louisiana bayou under a lily pad…I just mean checking around in smaller cities.

There's a big difference between the cost of surgery in Hollywood and the cost of surgery in Rochester, NY. Now, I know what you're thinking…"Yeah, but in Hollywood the doctors are better, right?" Not necessarily.

Take my favorite plastic surgery catastrophe, Michael Jackson. This guy has all the money in the world…he should be breathtakingly beautiful! In the dictionary next to the word "Gorgeous" they should have a picture of Michael Jackson, right? Well, here he is now left looking like a twisted, noseless freak. I can't believe he can get any children to even stay in the same room with him more-less into his bed. He's so scary looking!

With all that money he must have the best, most skilled plastic surgeons in the world, wouldn't you think? Then how in the world did they do that to his face??? Even if he begged them, "Please remove my nose and leave a cleft of bone with a little skin stretched over it," the best doctors in the world should have enough integrity to send the man to a psychiatrist…STAT!

My editorializing aside, the point is you can save upwards of a few thousand dollars in some cases just by seeking surgery in rural areas. Again, do your homework.

Go visit Grandma in Boise. While you're there go see a few surgeons, ask for references, and take a good look around their waiting rooms. That will tell you a lot. If the waiting room is full of eager patients…it's a good sign. Talk to them. Find out how they found him and if he's done any work on them before.

Talk to volunteers at the front desk of the local hospital. They get the dirt on everybody and they usually love to share. Word of mouth is powerful, and when people love a plastic surgeon they're happy to tell you about it.

But don't expect total candor (i.e. the truth about how they know this surgeon's work). They'll usually just tell you, 'He did great work on my friend (cousin, niece, etc.)' rather than, 'He did great work on my (insert droopy or bloated body part here).'

Like I said before, most happy plastic surgery veterans are not above lying a little to protect their own egos but they usually can't help but gush about a great doctor.

I know it sounds very simple, but most people never realize how much more expensive it is to have their surgery performed in a large city.

Yet another option to save some major cash is going to a teaching University hospital and letting some newbies operate on you. This option is only for the super-brave, but you have to believe that even though you may get a surgeon who's still wet behind the ears he's going to be working with great supervision of an experienced plastic surgeon, and you know they'll all be extra careful!

One of my readers wrote to me telling of her very good experience having liposuction, eyelid lift and breast augmentation performed at University of Cincinnati, OH Hand and Plastic Surgery Clinic.

Although this was 5 years ago, she said she spent only $2,500.00 and got good results. I can't tell you for sure how much it would cost today, but it may be worth looking into for those who are pinching every penny and aren't afraid of letting an inexperienced plastic surgeon operate on them.

Spanish Phrases to Know

These are just a few of the most important phrases you should know in Spanish if you are coming to the Dominican Republic for surgery (although they could come in handy in countless other situations, too!).

Do you speak English?

Tú hablas Inglés?

I have a headache.

Tengo un dolor de cabeza.

I have a stomachache.

Tengo un dolor de estómago.

My leg hurts.

Tengo dolor en mi pierna.

My legs hurt.

Tengo dolor en mis piernas.

My arm hurts.

Tengo dolor en mi brazo.

My arms hurt.

Tengo dolor en mis brazos.

My chest hurts.

Tengo dolor en mi pecho.

I need to throw up.

Necesito vomitar.

I need help.

Necesito ayuda.

I need to use the bathroom.

Necesito utilizar el baño.

Where is the bathroom?

Dondé esta el baño?

I want to brush my teeth.

Deseo cepillar mis dientes.

I'm cold.

Tengo frío.

I'm hungry.

Tengo hambre.

I'm thirsty.

Tengo sed.

I'm hot.

Tengo calor.

I feel sick.

Me siento enfermo.

May I have water?

Me das agua?

May I have juice?

Me das jugo?

My wound is bleeding.

Mi herida está sangrando.

And don't forget the most important two phrases…**Por Favor** (Please)
and **Gracias** (Thank You)!

List of Active Members of FILACP (Federacion Ibero Latinamericana de Cirugia Plastica y Reconstructiva) and Sociedad Dominicana de Cirugia Plastica y Reconstructiva in Domincan Republic

Plastic Surgeons in Santo Domingo

Abreu Montero, Jesus Dr
Centro de Cirugía Plastica y Lipoescultura
Calle Luis Amiama Tió #60, Arroyo Hondo
Santo Domingo
(809) 565-4261
Email: Jesús.abreu@verizon.net.do

Abreu Santana, Jose Ernesto Dr
Centro de Cirugía Plastica y Especialidades
Calle Manuel Maria Castillo #20
Santo Domingo
(809) 685-7250
Email: gisell_a@yahoo.com

Almonte Cruz-Ayala, Herman Dr
Centro Medico de la Universidad Central del Este
Residencia Uce III,
Avenida Pedro Henriquez Ureña #79
Santo Domingo
(809) 563-3667
Email: hermi_her@hotmail.com

Báez Comme, Ivanhoe F Dr
Centro de Cirugía Plastica y Especialidades
Calle Manuel Maria Castillo #20G
Santo Domingo
(809) 685-4906
Email: plastimed@hotmail.com

Cabral Guerrero, Héctor Dr
Instituto de Cirugía Especializada
Av Bolívar #208
Santo Domingo
(809) 685-4888

Carrasco, Ruben Dr
Centro de Cirugía Plastica Y Especialidades
Calle Manuel Maria Castillo #20G
Santo Domingo
(809) 686-1954
Email: carrasco@cirplastica.com

Carrón, José R Dr
Independencia 1061
Santo Domingo
(809) 686-2639
Email: jrcarron@hotmail.com

Cordero, Luis Andres Dr
Instituto de Cirugía Platistica
Calle Pedro A Lluberes #3
Santo Domingo
(809) 689-4322
Email: la.cordero@verizon.net.do

Crispin Luis Paulino Dr
Centro Medico Dominicano
Calle Luis F. Thomen #456, El Millon
(809) 531-0847

De La Cruz, Acosta Fernando Dr
Clínica Abreu
Calle Fabio Viallo #55
Santo Domingo
(809) 689-6115

De La Rosa, Saiz Quisqueya Dr
Centro Medico Real
Avenida Romulo Betancourt #215
Santo Domingo
(809) 687-3003

Encarnacion Bautista, Jose L
Centro de Fertilidad y Reproduccion Humana
Avenida Bolivar #405
Gazcue, Santo Domingo
(809) 221-0707
Email: drencarnan@hotmail.com

Espaillat Moya, Luis F Dr
Centro de Cirugia Plastica Espaillat
Guerra-Seijas
Calle Socorro Sanchez #56
Gazcue, Santo Domingo
(809) 412-7504

Espaillat, Lora Jose Dr
P A Lluberes 3
Santo Domingo
(809) 689-4322

Feliz Camilo, Katherine
Centro de Cirugia Plastica y Especialidades
Calle Manuel Maria Castillo #20G
Santo Domingo

González Valdez, Luis E Dr
S Sánchez 56
Santo Domingo
(809) 686-2417
Email: luisgonzalez@ciruplastic.com
Web Site (Hair Restoration) http://www.injerpelo.com
Web Site (Plastic Surgery) http://www.ciruplastic.com
***DOCTOR AND MORNING SECRETARY SPEAK ENGLISH**

Guashino Ginebra, Giancarlo Dr
Grupo Medico Naco
Calle Padre Fantino
Falco #12
Ensanche Naco, Santo Domingo
(809) 544-2972
Email: giancarlog3@hotmail.com

Guerra Seijas, Jose G Dr
Centro de Cirugia Plastica Espaillat
Guerra-Seijas
Calle Socorro Sánchez 56
Santo Domingo
(809) 412-7504

*Guerrero, Roberto Dr
PlastiCenter
Mustafa Kamal Atatuk #24
Santo Domingo
(809) 412-5035
(809) 616-1139
(809)343-7218
Email: ro.guerrero@verizon.net.do
Web Site http://www.guerreroplastic.com/
DOCTOR AND STAFF SPEAK ENGLISH

Guidicelli, Jean Paul Dr.
Centro de Cirugia Plastica Especialidades
Calle Manuel Maria Castillo #20G
Santo Domingo
(809) 689-8020

Herrand Perdomo, Hector A.
Centro de Cirugia Plastica y Especialidades
Calle Manuel Maria Castillo #20
Gazcue, Santo Domingo
(809) 689-2449
Email: h.herrand@verizon.net.do

Hernández Díaz, Mario Dr
Centro de Cirugia Plastica Internacional
Calle Camila Henriquez #25
Santo Domingo
(809) 530-4263

*Hernández Pizzoglio, Alejandro
PlastiCenter

Mustafa Kamal Atatuk #24
Naco, Santo Domingo
(809) 616-1015
(809) 412-5935
(809) 710-0605
Email: a.hernandez@verizon.net.do
Website: www.alejandrohernandez.com
DOCTOR AND STAFF SPEAK ENGLISH

Hernández López, Lourdes G Dra
G Godoy 8
Santo Domingo
(809) 686-6546

Hungría, José A. Dr.
Calle: Manuel Maria Castillo #20 Gazcue, Suite 105.
Santo Domingo
Tel. (809) 682-2683
Fax. (809) 221-5772
Email:hungria@cirplastica.com
Web Site: http://www.cirplastica.com/

Jiménez Miranda, Carlos Dr
Centro de Cirugia Integrada
Avenida Independencia #1061
Santo Domingo
(809) 689-8516
DOCTOR SPEAKS ENGLISH
(This is the surgeon who did my first two surgeries)

Lorenzo Ortiz, Guillermo Dr
Av 27 De Febrero
Santo Domingo
(809) 221-4050
Email:drg.lorenzo@verizon.net.do

Mallen, Nestor Tejada Dr
Centro De Ginecologia
Santo Domingo Norte
Calle Pedro Livio Cedeno #39
Santo Domingo

(809) 288-3522
Email: Nestormallen@hotmail.com

Marzan de Ramirez, Milady Dra.
Centro Medico Dominicano
Calle Luis F. Thomen #456
El Millon, Santo Domingo
(809) 537-5855

Medrano, Victor A. Dr
Centro Clinico Las Mercedes
No other information available

Mendez, Flerido Dr.
Centro de Cirugia Plastica y Especialidades
Calle Manuel Maria Castillo #20
Santo Domingo
(809) 685-7250
Email: dr.flerido@verizon.net.do

Mercedes Acosta, Severo Dr
Centro de Cirugia Plastica y Especialidades
Calle Manuel Maria Castillo #20
Santo Domingo
(809) 686-5826
Email: severo.m@verizon.net.do

Morales Pumarol, Ramón Dr
Centro de Cirugia Plastica Espaillat Guerra-Seijas
Calle Socorro Sánchez #56
Santo Domingo
(809) 688-5922

Munoz, Iberka Dr
Unidad de Cirugia Estetica y Reconstructiva
Calle Dr. Pineyro #101
Esq. Calle Julio Ortega
Santo Domingo
(809) 685-3766
Email: cuacua38@hotmail.com

Nieves, Andres Dr
Centro de Cirugia Integrada
Avenida Independencia #1061
Santo Domingo
(809)686-2730

Peña Encarnación, Julio C Dr
Centro de Cirugia Plastica y Especialidades
Calle Manuel Maria Castillo #20
Santo Domingo
(809) 685-8560
Email: Julio.pena@verizon.net.do

Rodriguez, Ramon A. Dr
Centro Medico San Pancracio
Calle 29 Este #1
Ensanche Luperon, Santo Domingo
(809) 684-1474

Schimensky, Kenneth Dr
Clinica de Cirugia Integrada
Avenida Independencia #1061
Santo Domingo
(809) 221-5601
Email: kschimensky@hotmail.com

Sesto A, Adolfo Dr
Clinica Corazones Unidos
Santo Domingo
(809) 563-0256
Email: asesto@tricom.net

Rubio, Nelson Dr
No other information available

Tapounet Brugal, Yira Dra
Centro de Cirugia Plastica y Especialidades
Calle Manuel Maria Castillo #20
Santo Domingo
(809) 689-2552

Ulerio, Hitler R. Dr
Clinica Union Medica
Suite 327
Avenida Juan Pablo Duarte #176
Santo Domingo
(809) 582-8282
Email: r.ulerio@verizon.net.do

Urena, Robert N Dr
Clinica Rodriguez Santos
Calle Bartolome Colon #20, Villa Consuelo
Santo Domingo
(809) 532-3925

Volquez, Petra Dra
Centro de Cirugia Plastica y Especialidades
Calle Manuel Maria Castillo #20
Santo Domingo
(809) 221-9465
Email: luisescano@verizon.net.do

PLASTIC SURGEONS IN SANTIAGO
Abreu Montero, Jesús M Dr
Rep de Argentina
Santiago
(809) 583-4510

Martínez, Emilio Dr
Av J P Duarte 176
Santiago
(809) 583-0938

Ulerio, Rafael Dr
Av J P Duarte 176
Santiago
(809) 582-8282

BARIATRIC SURGEONS/CLINICS IN SANTO DOMINGO
Dr. Luis Betances
Plaza de la Salud
Calle Pepillo Salcedo
Esq. Alturo Logroño
Ensanche la Fe,
Santo Domingo, Rep. Dom.
Tel.: 809.565.9989
FAX: 809.565.7925
Web Site: http://www.bariatrica.com

Cecilip
L A Tió 60
Santo Domingo
(809) 472-4548

Centro De Cirugía Plástica CxA
S Sánchez 56
Santo Domingo
(809) 686-0686

Centro De Cirugía Plástica
M M Castillo 20
Santo Domingo
(809) 686-7290

Centro De Cirugía Plástica
M M Castillo 20
Santo Domingo
(809) 686-7291

Centro De Cirugía Plástica CxA
S Sánchez 56
Santo Domingo
(809) 412-7529

Centro De Cirugía Plástica CxA
Residencia
Santo Domingo
(809) 530-3982

Centro De Cirugia Plastica Y Especialidades Santo Domingo Cecip
M M Castillo 20
Santo Domingo
(809) 686-7290

Centro De Cirugia Plastica Espaillat-Guerra Seijas Cxa
S Sánchez 56
Santo Domingo
(809) 686-0686

Clínica De Cirugía Integrada
Av Independencia 1061
Santo Domingo
(809) 689-7777

Clínica Jordan De Cirugía Plástica
Av Privada 6
Santo Domingo
(809) 482-7777
Email:dr.jordan@verizon.net.do

HOSPITALS AND CLINICS IN SANTIAGO
Clínica Corominas CxA
Restauración 57
Santiago
(809) 580-1171
Email:corominas@verizon.net.do

Centro Médico Cibao-Utesa, S A
Av J P Duarte 64
Santiago
(809) 582-6661

Sociedad Dominicana De Cirugia Plastica Y Reconstructiva, Inc.
M M Castillo 20
Santo Domingo
(809) 686-5826

Visit the Sociedad Dominicana de Cirugía Plástica y Reconstructiva web site:
http://filacp.org/espanol/miembros/santodomingo.htm

Sociedad Dominicana de Ortodoncia (Dominican Society of Orthodontists)
Visit: http://www.sdonet.org/default.htm

IN SANTO DOMINGO

Dra. Elizabeth Abud
Ave. 27 de Febrero # 481, Edif. Acuario
Tel: (809) 482-6738

Dr. Adolfo Arthur Nouel
Wenceslao Alvarez # 253, zona Universitaria
Tel: (809) 687-4149, 685-8657, 682-0503
Fax: (809) 221-4361
Email: adolfo@infocompu.com
Pagina Web: www.adolfo.arthur.net

Dr. Miguel Arthur Rodger
Wenceslao Alvarez # 253, zona Universitaria
Tel: (809) 687-4149, 685-8657, 682-0503
Fax: (809) 221-4361
Email:adolfo@infocompu.com
Pagina Web: www.adolfo.arthur.net

Dr. Eduardo Crespo
Ave. López De Vega # 33
Plaza Intercaribe Suite 216-A
Tel: (809) 563-2521
Email: eduardocrespo@verizon.net.do

Dr. Nildo De León
Paseo De Los Locutores # 22
Tel: (809) 622-5700

Dra. Patricia Defilló
Fantino Falco # 6
Edif. Profesional Corazones Unidos III
Tel: (809) 547-7005
Email: mpdefillo@hotmail.com

Dr. Luis R. Delgado R.
Abraham Lincoln, Plaza Lincoln J/42
Tel: (809) 227-6058, 472-0658
Email:luisdelgado_r@hotmail.com –or- delgado@verizon.net.do

Dr. Luis M. Despradel
Ave. Bolívar # 950, Apto 3-A
Tel: (809) 227-7127
Fax: (809) 567-8448

Dr. Luis Díaz Quero
Juan Isidro Jiménez # 7
Tel: (809) 689-9331

Dra. Dorhys Abrahim de Lockward
Prolongación Abraham Lincoln # 240
Arroyo Hondo
Tel: (809) 563-0831; Fax: (809) 541-8663

Dr. Julio Escoto
Ave. 27 de Febrero # 329
Evaristo Morales, Torre Elite, Suite 202
Tel: (809) 472-4605 Fax: 567-1374
Email: escoto.julio@verizon.net.do

Dr. Robert García
Luis F. Tomén # 110, Evaristo Morales
Torre Ejecutiva GAPO, Local 302
Tel: (809) 563-6954
Email: robertgacia25@hotmail.com

Dr. Francisco Garrido
Gustavo Mejía Ricart # 37
Edif. Boyero III, Suite 206
Tel: (809) 5471061
Email: garicorp@hotmail.com

Dra. Tania González
Jardinez del Embajador
Plaza Jardines del Embajador, Suite 310
Tel: (809) 508-3255

Dr. Rafael Hernández Bonnelly
Abraham Lincoln # 847
Edif. Profesional Lincoln Apto 2-A
Tel : (809)541-6788, Fax : (809)563-1249
Email: rhm@verizon.net.do
Email: rafael.hdez@verizon.net.do

Dr. Rafael Hernández Mota
Abraham Lincoln # 847

Edif. Profesional Lincoln Apto 2-A
Tel : (809)541-6788, Fax : (809)563-1249
Email: rhm@verizon.net.do
Email: rafael.hdez@verizon.net.do

Dr. Paul Lalane
Ave. Bolívar # 805, La Esperilla
Res. Plaza Bolívar Apto. G-104
Tel: (809) 687-4763

Dr. Milvio Linares
Ave. Pasteur # 107
Gazcue, Apartamento 102
Tel: (809) 687-1311

Dr. Julio Mejía
Luís F. Tomén # 110,
Torre Ejecutiva GAPO, Suite 206
Tel: (809) 472-4107
Email: julio.mejia@verizon.net.do

Dr. Tomas Morales Noboa
Abelardo Rodríguez Urdaneta # 8
2do piso, Gazcue
Tel: (809) 687-8627

Dra. María Isabel Núñez
Rafael Augusto Sánchez # 306
Plaza Intercaribe
Tel: (809) 547-1794

Dr. Franklin Ortega
Ave. Tiradentes # 30
Tel: (809) 549-7982
Fax: (809) 563-4996
Email: fbortega@hotmail.com

Dr. Alexis Ovalle
Ave. 27 de Febrero # 395
Suite 310, Plaza Quiqueya
Tel: (809) 566-5628
Email: aovalle14@hotmail.com

Dr. Claudio Pineda
Rafael Augusto Sánchez esq. López de Vega
Plaza Intercaribe Suite 303

Tel: (809) 563-3154 Fax: 563-3154
Email: claudiopinedarivera@yahoo.com

Dra. Nancy Puente
Ave. Bolívar # 755 esq. Máximo Gómez
Local 3ro
Tel: (809) 686-5994

Dra. Jacqueline Rodríguez Ramírez
Ave. 27 de Febrero # 329, Evaristo Morales
Torre Elite, Suite 202
Tel: (809) 472-4605
Fax: (809) 567-1374
Email: escoto.julio@verizon.net.do

Dr. Héctor Luis Rodríguez
Max Henríquez Ureña # 31
Ens. Naco
Tel: (809) 541-4146
Fax: (809) 541-3025
Email: ortoplan@verizon.net.do

Dr. Pavel Rodríguez
Gustavo Mejía Ricart
Edif. Boyero III, Suite 206
Tel: (809) 566-3608
Fax: (809) 547-1061
Email: vladimir.rquez@verizon.net.do

Dr. Milagros Ruíz
Lopez de Vega # 36
Plaza Intercaribe
Tel: (809) 683-2670
Email: milagros.r@verizon.net.do

Dra. Barbara Saladín
Jardines del Embajador
Plaza Jardines del Ambajador Suite 310
Tel: (809) 508-3255

Dra. Adela Santana
Ave. Bolívar # 950, apto 3-A
Tel: (809) 381-0870

Dra. Pilar Santana
Gracita Alvarez # 1
Tel: (809) 686-8919

Dr. Luis Serret Hernández
Ave. Bolívar # 755
Tel: (809) 689-3964

Dr. Francisco Socías
Abraham Lincoln # 502, 2do nivel
Tel: (809) 562-1710
Fax: (809) 472-1472
Email: franciscosocias@hotmail.com

Dr. Jose Luis Soto Perozo
Ave. Bolívar # 507
Tel: (809) 687-1032; (809) 686-0643
Email: laura.soto@verizon.net.do

Dra. María Soto
Ave. Bolivar esq. Máximo Gomez
Plaza Los Libertadores 2do, Local 9
Tel: (809) 686-1441

Dra. Maritza Yeb
Ave. Bolívar # 167
Tel: (809) 686-8292

IN SANTIAGO

Dra. Glennys Figueroa
José Ma. Cabral , Res. Los Colegios
Apto CMF, Tel: (809) 724-0079
Email: glennysf@yahoo.com

Dr. Richard Jiménez
Centro Comercial Las Trinitarias, Módulo 403
Juan Pablo Duarte esq. Maimón
Tel: (809) 582-1134
Email: r.jimenez2@verizon.net.do

Dr. Omar Marte
Calle 16 de Agosto
Edif. Julián Ramia Abaid, 2da pta
Tel: (809) 971-0222

Fax: (809) 241-4071
Email: omarmarte@verizon.net.do

Dra. Irys Núñez Taveras
Santiago Rodríguez # 36 (Altos)
Tel: (809) 971-3111
Email: y.nunez27@hotmail.com

Dra. Bexabeth Puig
Beller # 69 esq. Cuba
Tel: (809) 581-0964

Dra. Gladis Ramírez
E León Jiménez Edif. C-5, apto 12
Res. Los Girasoles
Tel: (809) 583 -5310
Fax: (809) 724-2600
Email: 117@hotmail.com

Dra. Rosanna Turbí
Ave. Rep. De Argentina
La Trinitaria, Edif. INCO
Tel: (809) 724-0354
Email:Rosannaturbi@hotmail.com

Dr. Fernando Valdéz Franco
12- A. Acevedo casi esq. Metropolitana
Los Jardines
Tel: (809) 247-4200
Fax: (809) 581-0179
Email:ferval@verizon.net.do

Dr. Gregory LLaverias Dunlop
calle restauracion No. 46 , esq. General Luperon
2do nivel santiago . Rep. Dominicana
Tels: (809) 583-0574
Fax (809) 971-0551
CEL: (809) 641-1122
Email:gllaverias@hotmail.com

In MAO

Dr. Saqib Khan
Clínica San Judas Tadeo
Calle Duarte # 54
Tel: (809) 572-7235
Email:saqibk@hotmail.com

In PUERTO PLATA

Dra. Bexabeth Puig
Beller # 69 esq. Cuba
Tel: (809) 686-5994

Dr. Saqib Khan
Calle Duarte # 75 Esq. Villanueva
Tel: (809) 586-6666
Fax: (809) 261-0499
Email:sagibk@hotmail.com

In MOCA

Dra. Iris Núñez
Santiago Rodríguez # 36
Tel: (809) 971-3111

Dr. Claudio Pineda
Moca, República Dominicana.
Tel: (809) 563-3154 ; Fax: 563-3154
Email:claudiopinedarivera@yahoo.com

In BONAO

Dr. Francisco Socías
Centro Odontológico Dra. Sang
16 de Agosto # 66
Tel: (809) 525-3264, fax: (809) 472-1472
Email:franciscosocias@hotmail.com

In LA ROMANA

Dr. Franklin Ortega
La Romana, República Dominicana.
Tel: (809) 549-7982; fax: (809) 563-4996
Email:fbortega@verizon.net.do
Email:fbortega@hotmail.com

Dr. Francisco Garrido
La Romana, República Dominicana.
Tel: (809) 5471061
Email:garicorp@hotmail.com

In SAN FRANCISCO DE MACORIS

Dr. Claudio Pineda
San Francisco de Macorís, República Dominicana.

Tel: (809) 563-3154 Fax: 563-3154
Email:claudiopinedarivera@yahoo.com

In LA VEGA

Dr. Luis M. Despradel
La Vega, República Dominicana.
Tel: (809) 573-3188

In JARABACOA

Dr. Luis M. Despradel
Jarabacoa, República Dominicana.
Tel: (809) 574-4552

PLASTIC SURGEONS OF COSTA RICA

Asociación de Costa Rica de Cirugía Plástica, Reconstructiva y Estética
Silvia Araya Matamoros
Presidenta
Apartado Postal 767- 3000
Heredia, COSTA RICA
Tel. 506 261 1914
Email: saraya@racsa.co.cr

Rodrigo Araya, M.D.
P.O. Box 12088 - 1000
San José, Costa Rica
Tel: (506) 297-0390
Fax: (506) 283-4296
Website: http://www.a-plastic-surgeon.com
Email: arayamd@a-plastic-surgeon.com

Cirujanos Plásticos S.A.
Paseo Colón, 1st. Avenue, 24th. and 26th. Streets
San José, Costa Rica
Telephone: (506) 223-7069 / (506) 222-6441
Fax: (506) 222-2520
Email:ctucan@sol.racsa.co.cr

Dr. Alejandro Lev
Torre Medica Paseo Colon Apartado 183-1007
San Jose, Costa Rica
(506) 221-8329
Web Site
http://www.edenia.com/medical/drlev.htm
Email: levplast@sol.racsa.co.cr

Rosenstock-Lieberman Center For Cosmetic Plastic Surgery at:
P.O. Box: 657-1005 San José, Costa Rica
Telephone: (506) 223-9933
U.S. Fax Number: (419) 844-2816
http://www.cosmetic-cr.com/
Email: info@cosmetic-cr.com

Dr. Jose Cohen

P.O. Box: 7-1540 - 1000, SAN JOSE - COSTA RICA
Phone: (506) 223-9933
Fax: (506) 223-9171
Web Site http://www.cosmetic-cr.com/josec/
Email:josec@cosmetic-cr.com

Arnoldo Fournier, M.D.
Santa Rita Hospital
8th Avenue, 15th-17th Streets, 2nd floor.
Phone: (506) 223-7214 / (506) 221-2225
Fax: (506) 255-4370
WebSite: http://www.drfournier.com/ing/index.html
Email: fournier@racsa.co.cr
DOCTOR SPEAKS ENGLISH

PLASTIC SURGEONS OF THAILAND

Dr. Paiboon CHITPRAPAI MD
Bangkok Hospital, Bangkok
Email: uro@bangkokhospital.com
http://www.bangkokhospital.com/english/uro/uro_sexchange.asp

Dr. Choomchoke JANWIMALUANG MD
Ban Don Hospital, Koh Samui
Email: info@sexchangeasia.com
http://www.srsthailand.com

Dr. Sirachai JINDARAK MD
Deja General Hospital, Bangkok
Email: deja_srs@sexchange-bangkok.com
http://www.sexchange-bangkok.com

Dr. Sanguan KUNAPORN MD
Phuket International Hospital, Phuket
Email: info@phuket-plasticsurgery.com
http://phuket-plasticsurgery.com

Dr. Kamol PANSRITUM MD
Bangkok Hospital, Bangkok
Email: info@mtfsurgery.com
http://www.mtfsurgery.com

Dr. Greechart PORNSINSIRIRAK MD
Yan Hee General Hospital, Bangkok
Email: info@yanhee.net
http://www.yanhee.net/serv_sexreass.htm

Dr. Bhumsak SAKSRI MD
Vibhavadi II Hospital, Bangkok
Email: bhumsak@thailandplasticsurgery.com
http://neopsc.com
Dr. Vichai SURAWONGSIN MD, Dr. Jirapong POONY MD
Pattaya International Hospital, Pattaya
Email: picpih@ptty.loxinfo.co.th
http://www.pattaya-inter-hospital.co.th/service.html

Dr. Preecha TIEWTRANON MD
Bangkok Nursing Home Hospital, Bangkok
Email: consult@pai.co.th
http://www.pai.co.th

Dr. Chettawut TULAYAPHANICH MD
Vibhavadi II Hospital, Bangkok
Email: info@chet-plasticsurgery.com
http://www.chet-plasticsurgery.com

Dr. Suporn WATANYUSAKUL MD
Aikchol Hospital, Chonburi
Email: contact@srs-thailand.com
http://srs-thailand.com

Board Certified Plastic Surgeons of Mexico
Asociacion Mexicana de Cirugia Plastica,Estetica y Reconstructiva
Email: mcper@cirugiaplastica.org.mx
Website: www.cirugiaplastica.org.mx

In ENSENADA
DR. ADRIAN
DIAZ CERON
(646) 176-02-95
Email: adc_surgery@hotmail.com

DR. ROBERTO
LAFARGA BALTAZAR
(646) 118- 67-50
(646) 118-67-55

DR. JOSE ANTONIO
MORALES GONZALEZ
(646) 178-78-38
(646) 178-28-04
Email: amorales@telnor.net

DR. MANUEL
NUÑEZ VIRGEN
(646) 176-36-82
(646) 176-39-40
Email: mnvirgen@hospitalguadalajara.com

DR. ROBERTO
PEREZ RANGEL
(646) 172-50-22
Email: dosaurio@telnor.net

In MEXICALI
DR. ADRIAN
AMEZCUA MANJARREZ C.
(686) 566-28-20
Email: manjarez@telnor.net

DR. JOSE
BARRAGAN CABRAL
(686) 555-63-01
(686) 552-21-17
Email: josebar@telnor.net

DR. COSME
CARDENAS BARO
(686) 553-55-57
(686) 553-55-48
Email: cosme@cosmetoplast.com

DR. GUSTAVO
GASPAR BLANCO
(686) 552-92-66
Email: drgaspar@telnor.net

DRA. NASTIA EUNICE
GONZÁLEZ AGUIRRE
(686) 582-35-60

DR. MARCO ANTONIO
GUTIERREZ LAMADRID
(686) 582-45-25
Email: toto_md@hotmail.com

DR. ADRIAN AMEZCUA
MANJARREZ CORTES
(686) 566-28-20
(686) 556-31-30
Email: manjarez@telnor.net

DR. ALEJANDRO
PAREDES VALLEJO
(686) 553-48-17
Email: alewalls@telnor.net

DR. MIGUEL A.
ROLON HERNANDEZ
(686) 553-56-56
(686) 553-58-28

DR. RODRIGO E.
VILDOSOLA ULLOA
(686) 554-03-84
(686) 552-29-29

In **ROSARITO**
DR. EDUARDO ULISES
GONGORA ALEJANDRE
(661) 231-61
Email: veek@telnor.net

In **TIJUANA**
DR. FRANCISCO
BUCIO MONTEMAYOR
(664) 686-4604
(664) 686-45-88
Ext. 22
Email: bucio@net-pla.net

DR. CARLOS
BUENROSTRO VAZQUEZ
(664) 634-11-77
(664) 634-03-09
Email:carlosbuen@cox.net

DR. JAIME
CALOCA ACOSTA
(664) 634-20-90
(664) 634-23-59
Email: drcaloca@drcaloca.com

DRA. MA. GUADALUPE
CARRILLO CISNEROS
(664) 686-55-99
Email: gcac@attglobal.net

DR. BERNARDO
CERVANTES SANCHEZ

(664) 684-72-50
(664) 621-85-23

DR. GASTON
DE LA GARZA MARTINEZ
(664) 686-48-66
(664) 686-51-56
(664) 681-86-46
Email: gaston@gtel.com.mx

DR. ORLANDO
FIGUEROA CERPA
(664) 634-69-90

DR. JUAN CARLOS
FUENTES AMEZCUA
(664) 634-19-03
Email:jcfa@telnor.net

DR. ARTURO
GONZALEZ MONTES
(664) 634-16-26
Email: art2rito54@hotmail.com

DR. HECTOR GUILLERMO
LINO ORTIZ
(664) 684-77-61
Email: drhectorlino@hotmail.com

DR. FERNANDO
LOUSTAUNAU CABALLERO
(664) 684-76-80
(664) 634-00-83
Email: luisfloustaunau@cox.net

DR. HECTOR MOISES
MILLA HINOJOSA
(664) 634-69-81
(664) 685-17-61

DR. GILBERTO
MONTFORT MARGAIN
(664) 684-09-58
(664) 684-18-93
Email: gilmont@telnor.net

DR. MANUEL
NUÑEZ VIRGEN
(664) 685-8662
(664) 685-9028
(664) 685-1900
Email: mnvirgen@hospitalguadalajara.com

DR. MIGUEL ANGEL
PARRA ESQUIVEL
(664) 681-73-48
Email: mparracpr@teleserviz.com
Email: m_angelp@hotmail.com

DR. JOSE ANTONIO
PEREZ HERNANDEZ
(664) 686-33-92

DR. ALEJANDRO
QUIROZ TEJEDA
(664) 634-19-03
(664) 634-1902

DR. MANUEL
RAMOS GALLO
(664) 681-26-29
Email: drmramos@bc.cablemas.com

DR. FERNANDO
ROBLES RODRIGUEZ
(664) 687-44-97
(664) 633-92-41
Email: rorfer1@yahoo.com.mx

DR. MARCO ANTONIO
RODAS RUIZ

(664) 684-17-13
(664) 634-10-25
Email: nefermarco@hotmail.com

DR. BENITO
RODRIGUEZ LOPEZ
(664) 634-23-07
(664) 634-23-08

DR. CARLOS J.
SALAZAR GARCIA-FIGUEROA
(664) 634-04-66
(664) 634-04-67

DR. JULIO
SALDAÑA ANGULO
(664) 634-22-08
(664) 634-73-68

DR. SERVANDO
SANDOVAL NUÑEZ
(664) 684-27-37
(664) 634-67-50

DR. SERGIO FERNANDO SOBERANES RIVERA
(664) 685-63-60
DR. LUIS
SUAREZ AVALOS
(664) 634-77-12
Email: luissuarezavalos@hotmail.com

DR. CAROLL
TOLEDO NADER
(664) 681-82-72
(664) 686-29-10
Email: toledo@cox.net

DR. JOSE LUIS
VALERO SALAS
(664) 684-25-51

Email: drluisvalero@hotmail.com
Email: valerol@telnor.net

DR. RICARDO
VEGA MONTIEL
(664) 686-55-99
(664) 686-62-02

DR. MARTÍN
YAÑEZ NAVARRO
(664) 686-55-99
Email: gyanavarro@yahoo.com

In LA PAZ
DR. ALFREDO
CARBALLO FIGUEROA
(612) 124-00-09
(612) 123-55-10
Email: alcafi@prodigy.net.mx

DR. FABIO
CASTRO ZARATE
(612) 124-04-00

DR. JOSUE HUMBERTO
VELARDE GALVEZ
(612) 123-44-03

DRA. JUDITH
YARHI CARRASCO
(612) 125-94-59
Email: drayarhi@hotmail.com

DR. JOSE LUIS
ZUÑIGA MENDOZA
(612) 122-96-29

In TAPACHULA
DR. CESAR A.
MOISES GALAN

(962) 625-64-48
(962) 623-02-35
Email: cliciper@hotmail.com

DR. CARLOS GMO.
OAXACA ESCOBAR
(962) 626-56-28
Email: droaxaca@prodigy.net.mx

In TUXTLA GUTIERREZ
DR. VICTOR MANUEL
ANZUETO ORTEGA
(961) 612-94-49
Email: cliciper@hotmail.com

DR. ERNESTO
COLINAS COSIO
(961) 612-06-70
Email: ecolinas@prodigy.net.mx

DRA. MA. ISABEL
FERRO MERAZ
(961) 614-27-93

DR. EDILBERTO
GARCIA SANTIAGO
(961) 611-46-26
(961) 614-75-49
Email: egarcias@latinmail.com

DR. FACUNDO JAVIER
PARADA OVALLE
(961) 602-81-55
(961) 602-81-58
(961) 602-80-18
Email: jparada@prodigy.net.mx

DR. MARIO CESAR
PAREDES ZENTENO

(961) 612-35-59
(961) 612-34-08
Email: dr_paredes@doctor.com

DR. IGNACIO
VAZQUEZ GOMEZ
(961) 614-28-30
Email: zivago2000@hotmail.com

DR.RICARDO
GONZALEZ RAMOS
(639) 472-8650

DR. ÁNGEL
ÁLVAREZ REGIL
(656) 623-2313
(656) 623-2310
(656) 618-3160
Email: juarezlazer@terra.com.mx

DR. CARLOS
ARCINIEGA SALCIDO
(656) 613-3709

DR. RAFAEL
FLORES CASTRO
(656) 615-2802
(656) 615-2803

DR. ALEJANDRO
GUERRERO REYES
(656) 687-1549
(656) 687-0908
Email: algrorey@hotmail.com

DR. RAYMUNDO
HOLGUIN MENESES
(656) 611-2222
     EXT. 350
Email: holguin_raymundo@latinmail.com

DR MIGUEL
NUTIS SHNAIDER
(656) 614-2074

DR. CARLOS
SOLANO MORALES
(656) 627-0788

DR. OSCAR
VILLARREAL GURROLA
(656) 618-1145
Email: vioscar@yahoo.com.mx

DR.HECTOR FCO.JAVIER
PERALTA PORRAS
(656) 616-7717
(656) 613-5620

In CHIHUAHUA
DR. RICARDO
BACA MARTINEZ
(614) 410-2159
Email: ricardobaca@hotmail.com

DR. JAIME ERNESTO
CHACON GONZALEZ
(614) 439-2792
DR. PABLO
CHAPA MEDELLIN
(614) 430-13-76
Email: cpr2020@prodigy.net.mx

DR. RENE XICOTENCATL
CHAVIRA SANTOS
(614) 439-2888
Email: rchavira@hospitalcima.com.mx

DR. NOEL
DEL VAL OCHOA
(614) 410-4175

Email: ndelval@mail.ep.com.mx

DR. JORGE
GALVAN ANTILLON
 (614) 413-1328
(614) 413-8822

DR. JORGE HUMBERTO
GARCIA ROMO
 (614) 415-1580
(614) 430-1717
Email: garciaromo_dr@hotmail.com

DR. GUILLERMO
MODESTO GONZALEZ
 (614) 413-0317
(614) 414-5929

DR. MIGUEL
NUTIS SHNAIDER
 (614) 614-2074

DR. ERNESTO RAUL
PAZ MURGA
 (614) 413-0279
Email: erpaz@att.net.mx

DR. PEDRO M.
RAMIREZ GODINEZ
 (614) 410-7540
(614) 415-9384

DR. MIGUEL ANGEL
SALGADO CASTILLO
(614) 426-6137
(614) 414-5275
(614) 413-9915
Email: masalgado66@aol.com

DR. ABEL
SEPULVEDA LARA
(614) 426-04-30

DR. ERNESTO
THEUREL SANGEADO
(614) 415-2660
(614) 415-2737
Email: theurell@cima-chihuahua.com.mx

DR. JESUS ALBERTO
TRIMMER HERNANDEZ
(614) 439-2761
Email: drjtrimmer@hotmail.com

DR. JOSE NAPOLEON
ZUÑIGA SANCHEZ
(614) 413-8484
Email: clinicaboticelli@yahoo.com.mx

In MONCLOVA
DR. JOSÉ ALEJANDRO
MEDINA TAMEZ
(866) 635-65-50

In SALTILLO
DR. RUFINO
IRIBARREN MORENO
(844) 485-01-18

DR. JESUS JOSE
JURADO GONZALES
(844) 416-79-20
(844) 415-67-20

DR. HERNAN
MARTINEZ LOPEZ
(844) 485-01-07
(844) 485-02-62
Email: hernanmtz@prodigy.net.mx

DR. JUAN JOSE
MENDEZ TREVIÑO
(844) 415-70-79
(844) 415-70-04
Email: j.j.mendez60@hotmail.com

In TORREON
DR. AGUSTIN ARTURO
BECERRIL PAZARAN
(871) 729-0440
(871) 727-4293

DRA. MA. DEL ROCIO
COLINAS ALVAREZ
 (871) 717-93-48
Email: rociocolinas13@hotmail.com

DR. VICTOR MANUEL
CORONA MEDINA
(871) 712-98-76
(871) 716-75-50
Email: drvictorcorona@hotmail.com

DR. JAVIER
DE LA PEÑA CORTES
(871) 718-33-11
Email: jdelapenac@hotmail.com

DR. LUIS GERARDO
ORNELAS REYNOSO
Email: luis_ornelas@yahoo.com

DR. JOSE LUIS
VILLARREAL MAIZ
(871) 721-22-11
(871) 721-33-32
Email: joseluis_vm@prodigy.net.mx

In Colima
DR. RAYMUNDO A.
COVARRUVIAS BERMEJO
(312) 312-50-98

In Mexico City
DR. OSCAR
ADAN RIVAS
(55) 5564-7815
Email: adanoscar@prodigy.net.mx

DRA. MARIA TERESA
AGUILAR IBARRA
(55) 5511-8017

DR. FERNANDO
AGUILAR MAYTORENA
(55) 5593-1080
Email: fdoam@prodigy.net.mx

DR. ALEJANDRO
ALARCON ROMERO
(55) 5363-73-41
Email: alexalarconr@axtel.net

DR. JOSE ANTONIO
ALEJANDRE SUAREZ
(55) 5564-7838

DR. JUAN ANGEL FELIX
ALTIMIR IÑESTA
(55) 5533-5560
(55) 5533-5561

DR. CARLOS DE JESUS
ALVAREZ DIAZ
(55) 5610-3431
Email: adcj@servidor.unam.mx

DRA. VANESSA DAYANA
ALVAREZ Y PEREZ
(55) 5395-0412
(55) 5395-0776
Email: vdayp@hotmail.com

DR. HUMBERTO
ANDUAGA DOMINGUEZ
(55) 5574-0067

DR. HECTOR
ANGULO ROMERO
(55) 5208-2904
Email: hearsince@hotmail.com

DRA. MARISELA
ANTILLON BUSTAMANTE
(55) 5574-6269
Email: antillon65@hotmail.com

DRA. A. M. ZAMIRA
APIS HERNANDEZ
(55) 5424-0472
(55) 5606-6222
ext. 4305
Email: zamiraapis@yahoo.com

DR. JOAQUIN
ARAICO LAGUILLO
(55) 5553-2517
(55) 5286-8451

DR. IGNACIO HECTOR
ARAMBULA ALVAREZ
(55) 5652-2200
(55) 5652-2222

DR. JORGE
ARELLANO ARREGUIN
(55) 5488-2222
Email: drjarreguin@yahoo.com
Email: jorgearreguin@yahoo.com.mx

DR. PABLO
ARIZTI GALNARES

(55) 5652-1543
(55) 5652-9775
Email: pabloarizti@aol.com

DR. JORGE
ATILANO MONTES DE OCA
(55) 5554-2045
(55) 5554-2184
Email: atilano_jorge@yahoo.com

DR. ROSENDO
AYALA GONZALEZ
(55) 5254-2686
Email: ayalarosendo@terra.com.mx

DR. EDUARDO
AYUSO RODRIGUEZ
(55) 5752-7602

DR. ALEJANDRO
AZUELA PINEDA
(55) 5520-3679
Email: drazuela@depilight.com.mx

DR. VICTOR HUGO
BAEZ GRANADOS
(55) 5553-2517
(55) 5286-8451

DR. BERNARDO
BALTAZAR
(55) 5574-6002
Email: bernanrdobaltazar@yahoo.com.mx

DR. MANUEL
BARRANTES TIJERINA
(55) 5272-2702
Email: eldoctor98@prodigy.net.mx

DR. MARIO
BARRIOS RIVERON

(55) 5543-3081
(55) 5669-1103

DR. MARIO
BECERRA CALETTI
(55) 5564-0800
Email: becerram@infosel.net.mx

DR. FEDERICO
BENITEZ LANDA
(55) 5564-0281
(55) 5574-3992
Email: cirplas@prodigy.net.mx

DR. FIDEL
BERLANGA RAMIREZ
Email: f_berlanga@att.net.mx

DRA. IRMA YOLANDA
BERNAL MARISCAL
(55) 5543-8470
Email: irma_y@hotmail.com

DR. GIOVANNI
BETTI KRAEMER
(55) 5246-9633
(55) 5202-8660
(55) 5202-9983
Email: drgiovannibetti@hotmail.com

DR. JAIME Y.
BOLIVAR FLORES
(55) 5666-8782
Email: ybolivar@yahoo.com

DR. LEONOR
BRAVO QUEZADA
(55) 5119-3027
(55) 5754-4447
ext. 538

DR. RAFAEL
BRIONES VELASCO
(55) 5568-5611
(55) 5652-8575
Email: rbrionesv@prodigy.net.mx

DRA. PATRICIA
BUTRON GANDARILLA
(55) 5528-7374
(55) 5515-1604

DR. EDUARDO S.
CABALLERO BARQUERA
(55) 1997-7900
(55) 1997-7901
Email: ecaba@axtel.net

DR. ALBERTO
CAHUANA QUISPE
(55) 5353-1452
(55) 5568-6854
(55) 5528-8422
Email: acqdoc@hotmail.com

DR. JAVIER AGUSTIN CARLOS
CAMACHO MONDRAGÓN
(55) 5652-2213
(55) 5568-9366
Email: javier_14140@yahoo.com

DRA. MA. ISABEL
CARAVANTES CORTES
(55) 5574-6266
(55) 5574-6269
Email: caravantes@infosel.net.mx

DR. ANGEL
CARRANZA MORALES
(55) 5682-8911
(55) 5682-8717

Email: carranza@cicer.com.mx

DR. FCO JAVIER
CARRERA GOMEZ
(55) 5208-7243
(55) 5533-1314
Email: jcarrerag@yahoo.com

DR. PEDRO FCO.
CEBALLOS MEDINA
(55) 5672-5284

DRA. MA.DEL PILAR
CEDILLO LEY
(55) 5515-3539
(55) 2614-2221

DR. JOSE JORGE
CELIO MANCERA
(55) 5333-2539
(55) 5207-4513
Email: jorgecelio@yahoo.com

DR. VICTOR S.
CHAVEZ ABRAHAM
(55) 5516-0794
(55) 5516-0795
Email: chavs65@prodigy.net.mx
Email: vicchavezabraham@yahoo.com.mx

DR. RICARDO
CIENFUEGOS MONROY
(55) 5574-8405
(55) 5265-1800
Ext. 4310
Email: rcienfuegos@usa.net

DR. ALEJANDRO
CORONA PADILLA
(55) 5250-0098
Email:dracorona@prodigy.net.mx

DR. FELIX
CORRAL MORALES
(55) 5543-3666
Email: felixcorral@hotmail.com

DR. ANGEL R.
CORZO SOSA
(55) 5517-9273
Email: angelcorzo@yahoo.com

DR. ALEJANDRO
CRESPO SCHMIDT
(55) 5135-2992
(55) 5135-2993
Email: alejandro@crespo.com

DR. CESAR
CRUZ CERON
(55) 5586-5135
(55) 5586-5136
Email: cesarcruzceron@internet.com.mx

DR. ROBERTO
CRUZ PONCE
(55) 5584-0866

DR. RAMON
CUENCA GUERRA
(55) 5250-1814
Email: cirplast@prodigy.net.mx

DR. JESUS
CUENCA PARDO
(55) 5514-2829
Email: jcuencap@aol.com

DR. MARCO ANTONIO
CUERVO VERGARA
(55) 5579-2693

DRA. CECILIA A.
CUESY RAMIREZ
(55) 5250-4002
(55) 5605-6695

DR. CARLOS
DAUMAS GIL DE PARTEARROYO
(55) 5254-0106
(55) 5250-6352
Email: daumasdr@hotmail.com

DR. RUBEN
DAVALOS OROZCO
(55) 5533-3327, 5511-40-00 Ext.186
Email: davalosruben@hotmail.com

DR. MANUEL FERNANDO
DE LA TEJERA GARCIA
(55) 5561-6896

DRA. XITLALI
DE SAN JORGE CARDENAS
(55) 5524 8573
Email: ciruplast@hotmail.com

DR. CARLOS
DEL VECCHYO CALCANEO
(55) 5264-2632
(55) 5264-2638
Email: cdelvecchyoc@hotmail.com

DR. JOSE NICOLAS
DOMINGUEZ CHAVEZ-CAMACHO
(55) 5271-2399
(55) 5271-7548
Email: edom@infosel.net.mx

DR. ALEJANDRO
DUARTE Y SANCHEZ
(55) 5687-8385
Email: drduartes@prodigy.net.mx

DRA. RAQUEL
EGUILUZ ORDOÑEZ
DR. RENE EUGENIO
ERREJON DIAZ
(55) 5559-9944
(55) 5575-5333
Email: errejondr@terra.com
Email: reneerrejond@aol.com

DR. JOSE
ESCAMILLA OLIVERA
(55) 5662-8007
(55) 5662-1757
Email:cirplas@yahoo.com

DR. PABLO
ESCOBAR BOURGET
(55) 5525-6473
(55) 5696-0777

DRA. DIANA DEL CARMEN
ESPINOSA GARCIA
(55) 5594-2203
(55) 5671-1266
Email: dianaeg@prodigy.net.mx

DRA. SILVIA
ESPINOSA MACEDA
(55) 5523-7909
(55) 5523-7850

DR. PAULO
FAJARDO JIMENEZ
(55) 5574-7120
(55) 5265-1800
EXT. 330
Email: polfjc4@aol.com

DR. JACOBO
FELEMOVICIUS HERMANGUS

(55) 5246-9715
(55) 5246-9716
(55) 5246-9717
Email: fele@data.net.mx

DR. MOISES JAIME
FERNANDEZ ZAMBRANA
(55) 5652-8987

DR. FRANCISCO E.
FERREIRA AGUILA
(55) 5523-2312
(55) 5523-2193
Email: drferreira54@hotmail.com

DR. ANTONIO
FUENTE DEL CAMPO
(55) 5568-4153
(55) 5290-1727
Email: afdelc@attglobal.net

DR. SAMUEL
FUENTES ARELLANO
(55) 5519-6756
Email: samuelfuentesa@aol.com

DR. SERGIO
FUNES CRAVIOTO
(55) 5574-0029
Email: sifunes@yahoo.com.mx

DR. ARTURO
GABILONDO ROJAS
(55) 5528-4033

DR. FAUSTINO
GALVEZ PEREZ
(55) 5568-4213
(55) 5568-4217
Email: faustogal@hotmail.com

DR. ENRIQUE
GARAVITO SALAZAR
(55) 5523-3999
Email: e_garavito@yahoo.com.mx

DR. JOSE SANTOS MARTIN
GARCIA CANO PEREZ
(55) 5543-3666

DR. SANTIAGO
GARCIA CASAS
(55) 5652-9775
(55) 5652-1543
Email: ucplastica@aol.com

DR. GERARDO
GARCIA CUERVO
(55) 5254-0346
(55) 5255-5670

DR. ENRIQUE
GARCIA MURRAY
(55) 5568-0986
(55) 5568-3187
Email: egamurray@avantel.net

DR. RAUL
GARCIA RAMIREZ
(55) 5250-6685
(55) 5250-6297
Email: garcia21@prodigy.net.mx

DR. JOSE
GARCIA VELASCO
(55) 5652-9775
(55) 5652-1543
Email: ucplastica@aol.com

DR. RICARDO
GARFIAS CAMPOS

(55) 5276-2812
(55) 5616-9900
Ext. 556
Email: iuo@prodigy.net.mx

DR. HECTOR
GARIBAY RODRIGUEZ
(55) 5543-3666
(55) 5536-1095
Email: hegaro65@hotmail.com

DR. ROMAN
GARZON LOYO
(55) 5568-6921
(55) 5568-3334
Email: garzonr@mx.inter.net

DR. LUIS
GOMEZ CORREA
(55) 5593-1693

DR. JOSE G.
GONZÁLEZ MARTÍNEZ
(55) 5579-5831

DRA. MA. ELVIRA
GONZALEZ RAMIREZ
(55) 5135-1472
(55) 5135-1473
Email: maelglez@yahoo.com

DR. JORGE
GONZALEZ RENTERIA
(55) 5687-0769
(55) 5554-1108

DR. ANGEL
GONZALEZ RODRIGUEZ
(55) 5255-4492
Email: agr1929@msn.com

DR. JOSE LUIS
GONZALEZ VERDIGUEL
(55) 5265-2909

DR. GUSTAVO
GONZALEZ ZALDIVAR
(55) 5264-6807
(55) 5574-9105
Email: ggonzalez@direct.com.mx

DR. JORGE LUIS
GORTAREZ MARTINEZ
(55) 5564-1129
(55) 5574-4277
Email: gortarezjorge@hotmail.com

DR. PEDRO
GRAJEDA LOPEZ
(55) 5219-1419
(55) 5219-1519
Email: drpedrograjeda@hotmail.com

DR. RAUL
GRANADOS MARTINEZ
(55) 5568-5868
(55) 5652-3011
Ext. 4816
Email: raulgranados@mexis.com

DR. RODOLFO
GUERRERO PEREZ
(55) 5652-1543
(55) 5652-9775
Email: ucplastica@aol.com

DR. ROBERTO
GUTIERREZ CARMONA
(55) 5135-1432
(55) 5135-1433

DRA . VERONICA
GUTIERREZ GARCIA
(55) 5272-1508
(55) 5272-1309
Email: verogg@avantel.net

DRA. CLAUDIA
GUTIERREZ GOMEZ DE DEL HIERRO
(55) 5665-4907
(55) 5606-6222
Ext. 4329
Email: clauggdelh@yahoo.com.mx

DR. EDUARDO
GUTIERREZ SALGADO
(55) 5630-7383
Email: egut@doctor.com

DR. JOSE LUIS
HADDAD TAME
(55) 5202-8660
(55) 5202-8023
Email: hatame5@prodigy.net.mx

DR. CALIXTO
HARADA PRIETO
(55) 5516-7880
(55) 5516-4309
Email: haradacalix@yahoo.com

DR.JOSE HUGO
HERNANDEZ GARDUÑO
(55) 5684-5279
(55) 5265-2986
Email: cphugoh@avantel.net

DRA. IRENE
JARQUIN LOPEZ
(55) 5679-2751

DR. FRANCISCO HERNANDEZ
JIMENEZ
(55) 5602-7407

DR. RUBEN
HERNANDEZ ORDOÑEZ
(55) 5690-4264

DRA FANNY E.
HERRAN MOTA
(55) 5511-0444

DR. PABLO
HIDALGO-MONROY PORTILLO
(55) 5682-8174
(55) 5682-7964
Email: phmp@prodigy.net.mx

DR. OCTAVIO
HOYER PEREZAMADOR
(55) 5523-9298
(55) 5523-2371
(55) 5523-1223
Email: hoyer@terra.com.mx

DR. LUIS
IBARRA DIAZ
(55) 5533-5560
(55) 5533-5561
(55) 5511-8546

DR. MARTIN
IGLESIAS MORALES
(55) 5568-4356
(55) 5568-4357
Email: martiniglesias@infosel.net.mx

DR. SERAFIN M.
IGLESIAS VEGA
(55) 5545-2574
(55) 5250-5191

Email: s_iglessias@terra.com.mx

DR. FEDERICO
IÑIGO MUÑOZ
(55) 5286-7727
(55) 5211-6397
Email: iceger@prodigy.net.mx

DR. PEDRO JOSE
JAIDAR MATALOBOS
(55) 5606-8183
(55) 5606-6372
Email: pjjaidar@yahoo.com

DR. LUIS
JANEIRO BARROS
(55) 5562-1072
(55) 5562-1172
Email: drluisjaneiro@aol.com

DR. YUSEF
JIMENEZ MURAT
(55) 5606-2277, ext. 4326
Email: yusmd@prodigy.net.mx

DR. JOSE FRANCISCO
JIMENEZ REYNA
(55) 5670-0290
(55) 5646-5876
Email: jimreyna@prodigy.net.mx

DR. JORGE E.
KRASOVSKY SANTAMARINA
(55) 5514-9896
(55) 5514-9602
Email: jkrasovsky@hotmail.com

DR. SERGIO MIGUEL
KURT ROJAS
(55) 5553-8672
Email: sergiokurt@hotmail.com

DR. JOSE ALEJANDRO
LABORDE BADILLO
(55) 5255-4789
Email: labordealex@yahoo.com

DR. GUSTAVO
LEDEZMA RUBIO
(55) 5271-8999
(55) 5271-8001
ext.206

DR. ABRAHAM
LEISOREK RAPOPORT
(55) 5250-1905
(55) 5203-1385
Email: aleisore@avantel.net

DR. JOSE ANTONIO
LEON PEREZ
(55) 5516-2367
(55) 5516-2339
Email: leonv@prodigy.net.mx

DR. MIGUEL
LOMAS FUENTES
(55) 5542-6501
Email: miguel_lomas_fuentes@hotmail.com

DRA. DIANA PATRICIA
LOPEZ GARCIA
(55) 5254-4040
(55) 5531-3120
Email: dra_dianalopez_plastica@yahoo.com

DR. HOMERO
LOPEZ MONJARDIN
(55) 5514-5577
Email: homerolopez@yahoo.com

DR. LUIS ENRIQUE
LOZANO DUBERNARD
(55) 5559-9779
Email: lozduber@hotmail.com

DR. SERGIO
LOZANO TELLEZ
(55) 5606-5355
(55) 5246-9661
Email: cucaloz@yahoo.com

DR. IGNACIO
LUGO BELTRAN
(55) 5286-3109

DR. FDO. SERGIO
LUJAN OLIVAR
(55) 5564-0715

DR. FERNANDO
MAGALLANES NEGRETE
(55) 5272-2210
(55) 5246-9570
Email: fmagallanes@terra.com

DR. MIGUEL ANGEL
MALDONADO BERNAL
(55) 5586-0886
(55) 5586-9310
Email: miguelmaldonadober@yahoo.com.mx

DR. ERNESTO
MALDONADO GARCIA
(55) 5530-1167
Email: dremg@hotmail.com

DR. RICARDO
MALDONADO RUELAS
(55) 5264-2632
(55) 5264-2638

DR. GERARDO
MANUELL LEE
(55) 5575-6896
Email: manuellger@hotmail.com

DR. MARTIN
MANZO HERNANDEZ
(55) 5081-8100
Ext. 8203
Email: picoman@data.net.mx

DR. MARCO ANTONIO
MARIN RAMIREZ
(55) 5369-7524
Email: contab1@prodigy.net.mx

DR. CUAUHTEMOC
MARQUEZ ESPRIELLA
(55) 5528-8422
Email: temoc_2@hotmail.com

DR. MIGUEL
MARQUEZ DUPOTEX
(55) 5514-6297
(55) 5511-6649

DR. ALFONSO
MASSE SANCHEZ
(55) 5568-9366
(55) 5652-9689
(55) 5652-2011
Email: amassecpr@yahoo.com.mx

DR. JOSE
MAYA BEHAR
(55) 5272-2462
Email: josemaya@acnet.net

DR. MIGUEL ANGEL
MENDEZ FERNANDEZ

(55) 5606-8458
Email: drmendez@plasticsurgeryredding.com

DR. MARIO
MENDOZA ARELLANES
(55) 5652-9398

DR. MARIO
MENDOZA MUÑOZ
(55) 5606-7752
(55) 5528-3335
Email: mariomz@hotmail.com

DR. ALFREDO
MEZA PEREZ
(55) 5264-2632
(55) 5264-2638
Email: mezaper@prodigy.net.mx

DR. ADOLFO
MIRANDA VENCES
(55) 5615-4060

DR. SANTIAGO
MOLINA VELEZ
(55) 5674-4311
Email: santiagomolina2@yahoo.com

DR. FERNANDO
MOLINA MONTALVA
(55) 5568-4649
(55) 5652-8987
Email: qsussie4@yahoo.com.mx
Email: fermomo57@hotmail.com

DR. MANUEL
MONDRAGON DOMINGUEZ
(55) 5568-6695
(55) 5652-2330
Email: drmmd@prodigy.net.mx

DRA. S. CLAUDIA
MONTOYA GARCIA
(55) 5564-7965
(55) 5528-4489
Email: clumontoyamx@hotmail.com
Email: asclaudia@correoweb.com

DRA. MA. DEL CARMEN
MORENO ALVAREZ
(55) 5606-2777
(55) 5606-6222 Ext. 4430/4423

DRA. CARMEN
MORENO VERA
Email: carmorv@hotmail.com

DR. ALEJANDRO
MOYA LEIJA
(55) 5202-0289
(55) 5202-0180

DRA. ALICIA
MUÑOZ DE GRAY
(55) 5282-0302
(55) 5280-2242
 Email: draliciagray@aol.com

DR. MARIO EDUARDO
NAVARRETE RIVERA
(55) 5598-2111
(55) 5598-0794
Email: cirplastic@dr.com.mx

DRA REYNA
NERI CAZARES
(55) 55647814
(55) 5265-1800
Ext. 4610
Email: mgardu@avantel.net

DR. RAFAEL
NIETO MALDONADO
(55) 5588-9660
(55) 5588-1355
Email: rafanima@mixmail.com

DR. ENRIQUE
OCHOA DIAZ LOPEZ
(55) 5553-8672
(55) 5553-8959

DR. FRANCISCO XAVIER
OJEDA CASTAÑEDA
(55) 5255-4797
(55) 5255-4492
Email: oxeda@prodigy.net.mx

DR. EDUARDO
OLIVARES CASTRO
(55) 5514-0238
(55) 5511-3089
Email: eolivarescastro@yahoo.com.mx

DR. VICTOR
OLIVERA ZAVALETA
(55) 5393-7115

DR. ALVARO
OLMEDO ZORRILLA
(55) 5568-2130
(55) 5568-2524
Email: aolmedoz@hotmail.com

DR. PAUL JAY
OLSOFF PAGOVICH
(55) 5515-3639
(55) 5271-2255
Email: paulolsoff@aol.com

DR. JORGE RENE
OROPEZA MORALES

(55) 5208-7243
(55) 5533-1314
(55) 5265-2909
Email: joropeza@prodigy.net.mx
Email: oropeza@cirugiaplastica.org.mx

DR. FERNANDO
ORTIZ MONASTERIO
(55) 5652-8987
(55) 5568-4649
Email: fortizm@prodigy.net.mx

DR. LUIS
ORTIZ OSCOY
(55) 5520-5811
(55) 5520-1493
Email: rodin@mail.internet.com.mx

DR. RICARDO CESAR
PACHECO LOPEZ
(55) 5264-2632
(55) 5264-2638
Email: rpache@netmex.com

DRA. GUILLERMINA
PADILLA PEÑA
(55) 5271-0378
Email: menelik@prodigy.net.mx

DR. EDGARDO
PALACIO LOPEZ
(55) 5586-4940
(55) 5752-1234
Email: drpalacio@hotmail.com

DR. ANGEL
PAPADOPULOS ESCOBAR
(55) 5574-1473
(55) 5574-6589
Email: angel_papadopulos@tutopia.com

DR. SAMUEL
PARADA VILLAVICENCIO
(55) 5246-9570

DRA. ESPERANZA
PAREDES MONDRAGON
(55) 5604-3926
(55) 5590-5938

DR. JAVIER
PEDROZA AGUAYO
(55) 5580-5259
(55) 5395-8569

DR. JOSE LUIS
PEREZ AVALOS
(55) 5264-6807

DRA. ARACELI
PEREZ GONZALEZ
(55) 5568-4217
Email: arapeli@podernet.com.mx

DR. ENRIQUE
PIÑA MORA
(55) 5265-2919
(55) 5265-2900
Ext. 2419
Email: pinamora@hotmail.com

DR. JORGE ALBERTO
PORTER ROBLES
(55) 5543-3666
(55) 5536-1095
Email: porterobles@hotmail.com

DR. RAYMUNDO BENJAMIN
PRIEGO BLANCAS
(55) 5540-20-60
(55) 5511-33-85
Email: priego@microcirugiaymano.com.mx

DR. ANGEL
PUENTE SANCHEZ
(55) 5545-3754
Email: puentehervella@prodigy.net.mx

DR. JOSE ULISES
QUEVEDO DESCHAMPS
(55) 5564-4098
(55) 5584-7567
Email: uli_cirujano_plastico@hotmail.com

DR. MARIO
QUIJANO HERNANDEZ
(55) 5292-5688
(52) 5292-5639
Email: mquijanoh@yahoo.com

DR. ERNESTO A.
RAMIREZ LOZANO
(55) 5254-6723
Email: dreramirezl@prodigy.net.mx

DRA. SILVIA
RAMIREZ TEJEDA
(55) 5679-3061
Email: sramirezt@tutopia.com

DR. LUIS ERNESTO
RAMOS DURON
(55) 5575-1776
Email: lramos@gsm.pemex.com

DR. HERIBERTO
RANGEL GASPAR
(55) 5574-7633
(55) 5264-0127
Email: hrangelg@yahoo.com

DR. JUAN CARLOS
RENTERIA COVARRUBIAS

(55) 5273-1651
(55) 5273-1049
Email: rentcov7@msn.com
Email: rentcov7@prodigy.net.mx

DR. FRANCISCO F.
REYES JACOME
(55) 5559-0103

DR. ALBERTO
REYES PARRAGA Y
TELLO DE MENESES
(55) 5523-4192

DR. LUIS ANTONIO
REYES QUIJANO
(55) 5590-1147
(55) 5579-6042
Email: dreyesquijano@starmedia.com

DR. AGUSTIN
REYES ROMERO
(55) 5568-6909
(55) 5652-3011
Ext. 4747

DR. RAFAEL
REYNOSO CAMPO
(55) 5652-8271
(55) 5652-8414
Email: mail@cicer.com.mx

DR. JAVIER
RIVAS JIMENEZ
(55) 5514-7430
Email: doctorjavierrivas@yahoo.com

DR. BERNARDO
RIVAS LEON
(55) 5652-9395
Email: berba@prodigy.net.mx

DRA. MA. TERESA
RIVAS TORRES
(55) 5549-7227
(55) 5652-2222
Email: tererivas@yahoo.com

DRA. MA. DEL PILAR
RIVERA
(55) 5574-0067
Email: dra_rivera_ciruplastica@hotmail.com

DR. JUAN PEDRO
ROBLES LÓPEZ
(55) 5584-5511
Email: grupomedcomsc@prodigy.net.mx

DR. DANIEL
RODRIGUEZ ALVAREZ
(55) 5589-6035

DR. ENRIQUE
RODRIGUEZ PATIÑO
(55) 5554-7592
Email: erodriguezpat@msn.com

DRA. LOURDES DEL CARMEN
RODRIGUEZ RODRIGUEZ
(55) 5265-2909
Email: lulurrod@hotmail.com

DRA. ELIZABETH DEL C.
RODRIGUEZ ROJAS
(55) 5697-2834
Email: elirodri@prodigy.net.mx

DR. ORBELIN
ROJAS ALVAREZ
(55) 5586-3313

DRA. ADRIANA P.
ROJO BLANCO

(55) 5652-8987
Email: laserend@prodigy.net.mx

DR. MIGUEL
ROLON HERNANDEZ
(55) 5280-0723
(55) 5553-5828
Email: doctor_rolon@hotmail.com

DR. JOSE LUIS
ROMERO ZARATE
(55) 5584-8344
Email: jlromeroz@terra.com

DR. RAMON H.
ROSADO CASTRO
(55) 5520-3679
Email: drrosado@depilight.com.mx

DR. IVAN AUGUSTO
ROSALES BERBER
(55) 5606-97-43 / 56-06-22-77 EXT. 4446
Email: iarv@prodigy.net.mx

DRA. LUCERO
RUBIO ARIAS
(55) 5208-0423
(55) 5538-5592
Email: lucess00@hotmail.com

DR. HECTOR HORACIO
SALCIDO CALZADILLA
(55) 5534-2081
Email: hectorsalcido@yahoo.com

DR. DANIEL JULIAN
SAN MARTIN CHAVEZ
(55) 5273-5833
(55) 5273-8645
Email: surgery2@hotmail.com
Email: surgery@cablevision.net.mx

DR. JESUS L.
SANCHEZ BUENDIA
(55) 5574-3787
(55) 5211-7873

DR. JORGE
SANCHEZ DE LA BARQUERA RAMOS
(55) 5584-3332
(55) 5264-1412

DR. XAVIER ANTONIO
SANCHEZ GARCÍA
(55) 5424-2394
Email: drsanchez@prodigy.net.mx

DRA. LAURA
SANCHEZ VILORIA
(55) 5543-3666
Email: vil_san@yahoo.com

DR. RAFAEL
SANDOVAL GARCIA
(55) 5674-1372
(55) 5672-9102
Email: ces@prodigy.net.mx

DRA. MA. ELENA
SANDOVAL OCHOA
(55) 5568-5891
Email: meso22@prodigy.net.mx

DR. CESAR DE JESUS
SANTIAGO LANDA
(55) 5264-1214
(55) 5574-1010
(55) 5265-1800
Ext. 330
Email: sanland@prodigy.net.mx

DRA. BEATRIZ E.
SANTILLAN AGUIRRE
5533-3327 / 5511-40-00, Ext.186 - 124
Email: bsantillan@prodigy.net.mx

DR. ALFONSO
SANTOS TORRES
(55) 5264-6899
Email: santos_alfonso@hotmail.com

DR. NICOLAS
SASTRE ORTIZ
(55) 5208-5426
(55) 5514-6484
Email: dr_nicolassastre@hotmail.com

DR. ALFONSO
SERRANO REBEIL
(55) 5570-7032

DR. ISAAC
SHTURMAN SIROTA
(55) 5395-0412
(55) 5395-0776
Email: corpo_re@yahoo.com

DRA. TERESITA
SILVA DIAZ
(55) 5564-0800

DR. JORGE
SOLA VALDES
(55) 5652-2222
(55) 5652-0000
Email: pilobon@prodigy.net.mx
Email: sola@cirugiaplastica.org.mx

DR. CHARBEL ANDRES
SOSA AZAR
(55) 5575-4708
Email: charbelps@yahoo.com

DR. ARTURO
SUAREZ COLIN
(55) 5264-0127
(55) 5574-7633
Ext. 331

DR. CLEMENTE RAFAEL
SUAREZ MENENDEZ
(55) 5271-89-99
(55) 5271-80-07
(55) 5611-52-14
Email: f1953@prodigy.net.mx

DRA. IRENE
TALAMAS VAZQUEZ
(55) 5575-2474
(55) 5575-2465

DR. JOSE
TELICH VIDAL
(55) 5568-6849
Email: drtelich@df1.telmex.net.mx

DR. RAYMUNDO
TORRES PIÑA
(55) 5264-2638
(55) 5264-2632
Email: torres_cirplast@hotmail.com

DR. SILVERIO
TOVAR ZAMUDIO
(55) 5639-2820
(55) 5639-2829
Email: silverio_tovar@hotmail.com

DR. JUAN ANTONIO
TREVIÑO MACIAS
(55) 5523-1077
(55) 5687-0592

Email: trevi334@hotmail.com
Email: trevi334@yahoo.com.mx

DR. IGNACIO
TRIGOS MICOLO
(55) 5511-0444
Email: itrigos@hotmail.com

DR. JORGE
TRUJILLO GONZALEZ
(55) 5543-2550
Email: docky9@hotmail.com

DR. JUAN ANTONIO
UGALDE VITELLY
(55) 5208-8575
Email: ugalde.juanantonio@corrreoweb.com

DR. FERNANDO
URRUTIA GONZALEZ
(55) 5575-1325
(55) 5559-0753
Email: doctorfernandourrutia@hotmail.com
Email: olindasa@mail.internet.com.mx

DR. SERGIO
URRUTIA RUIZ
(55) 5575-1325
(55) 5575-3252
(55) 5575-3257

DR. JOSE LUIS
VALDÉS GALICIA
(55) 5219-1419
(55) 5219-1518
(55) 5584-3962
Email: jlvaldes@cirugiaplastica.org.mx

DR. RAUL ALFONSO
VALLARTA RODRIGUEZ

(55) 5528-4489
(55) 5606-2277,
ext..4328
Email: vallacom@prodigy.net.mx

DR. VLADIMIR
VAZQUEZ AMBRIZ
(55) 5652-8993
(55) 5652-9798
Email: vva7@prodigy.net.mx

DR. ALFREDO
VAZQUEZ CARRILLO
(55) 5273-4123
Email: avazquez@iwm.com.mx

DR. RODOLFO OTHON
VAZQUEZ GONZALEZ
(55) 5276-2763
Email: othon@avantel.net

DR. ALFONSO
VEGA RODRIGUEZ
(55) 5652-8779
(55) 5652-3585

DR. MA. LUISA
VELASCO VILLASEÑOR
(55) 5514-3214
(55) 5514-3453
Email: maluvelascomx@yahoo.com.mx

DR. JACOBO
VERBITZKY BORKOW
(55) 5271-7188
Email:jacoboverbitzky@hotmail.com

DR. MIGUEL EVARISTO
VIERA NUÑEZ
(55) 5574-5033
(55) 5264-8886

Email: 14876@digitel.net.mx

DR. JAVIER
VILCHIS LICON
(55) 5516-8313
(55) 5278-2300
Ext. 2201
Email: drjvilchis@hotmail.com

DR. EVARISTO
VILLALOBOS GARCIA
(55) 5549-8655

DR. DONALDO
VILLALOBOS LOPEZ
(55) 5359-4424

DR. MARTIN
VILLASEÑOR BAZALDUA
(55) 5557-5083
(55) 5557-3100

DR. ENRIQUE
VINAGERAS GUARNEROS
(55) 5687-9206
(55) 5536-3564

DR. SERGIO
ZENTENO ALANIS
(55) 5523-9200
(55) 5536-0686
Email: ezenteno@cisco.com

DR. JAVIER
ZEPEDA RODRIGUEZ
(55) 5531-9530
(55) 5531-9531
Email: jzepeda245@yahoo.com.mx

DR. MARIA BEATRIZ
ZEVALLOS CORDOVA

(55) 5574-8724
(55) 5265-1800
Ext. 4725
Email: bzevallos68@msn.com

Members of the International Society of Aesthetic Plastic Surgery

ANNANDALE Zacharias F., MD
Box 11694, Silver Lakes
Pretoria 0054
Tel. 27-12-807-2695 / 27-12-807-2696
SOUTH AFRICA
Email: zfa@medi.co.za

BERKOWITZ Leslie, MD
PO Box 785129
Sandton 2146
Tel. 27-11-884-4419 / 27-11-884-6766
SOUTH AFRICA
Email: lesb@global.co.za

BRAUN Saul A., MD
PO Box 52828
Saxonwold, 2132
Tel. 27-11-788-4956 / 27-11-788-5724
SOUTH AFRICA
Email: info@drbraun.co.za

CHING Vernon, MD
Linksfield Park Clinic
Council Road Linksfield
Tel. 27-11-485-3393 / 27-11-485-3394
Email: vchingps@global.co.za
SOUTH AFRICA

COOKE John L., MD
411 Currie Road
Durban 4001
Tel. 27-31-207-6977 / 27-31-207-6978
SOUTH AFRICA
Email: cooke@ionet.co.za

FAYMAN Moshe S., MD
PO Box 1708

Parklands 2121
Tel. 27-11-788-1503/442-4545
27-11-788-6090
SOUTH AFRICA
Email: fayman@iafrica.com

FERNANDES Desmond Brian, MD
822 Fountain Medical Centre
Heerengracht 8001
Tel. 27-21-425-2310 / 27-21-418-1113
SOUTH AFRICA
Email: des@environ.co.za

FORD Thomas Dominic, MD
PO Box 130891
Gauteng
Tel. 27-011-4631210 / 27-011-4632485
Bryanston 2074
SOUTH AFRICA
Email: tomford@pixie.co.za

GORDON Luke, MD
Glynnwood Medical Suites
Suite 202
Tel. 27-11-421-8486 / 27-11-421-8449
Benoni 1500
Email: lgordon@icon.co.za
SOUTH AFRICA

JOHANNES Siegmund, MD
PO Box 87140
Houghton 2041
Tel. 27-11-462-7475 / 27-11-462-7424
SOUTH AFRICA
Email: sjohannes@infodoor.co.za

LAMONT Alastair, MD
PO Box 3072
Halfway House 1685
Tel. 27-11-3101724 / 27-11-3101861
SOUTH AFRICA

Email: lamonta@iafrica.com

LAZARUS Dirk, MD
822 Fountain Medical Centre
Cape Town 8001
Tel. 27-21-425 3580 / 27-21-418 1113
SOUTH AFRICA
Email: dirk@shirnel.com

MIDDELHOVEN Hans, MD
PO Box 263597
Three Rivers Vereeniging
Tel. 27-16-455-1664 / 527-16-422-0711
1935
Email: mwjmid@mweb.co.za
SOUTH AFRICA

MORRIS Warwick M. M., MD
201 Parklands Medical Centre
Hopelands Road
Tel. 27-31-209-5422 / 27-31-209-5422
Durban 4001
Email: morriswm@mweb.co.za
SOUTH AFRICA

MORRISON Gavin, MD
209 Newlands Surgical Clinic
Claremont 7700
Tel. 27-21-683-9220 / 27-21-683-9226
SOUTH AFRICA
Email: morrison@netactive.co.za

NICHOLSON Roger David, MD
Suite 206A Sandton Clinic
PO Box 3974
Tel. 27-11-706-7978 / 27-11-463-6007
Cramerview 2060
Email: rogernic@netactive.co.za
SOUTH AFRICA

NIKSCHTAT Heinrich, MD

PO Box 3766
Bloemfontein, 9300
Tel. 27-51-444-3757
SOUTH AFRICA
Email: gnpcit@mmed.uovs.az.za

POTTIE Rodger, MD
PO Box 39750
Moreleta Park, Pretoria 0040
Tel. 27-12-998-8995/6 27-12-998-8998
SOUTH AFRICA
Email: rodgerpottie@bitcc.co.za

PRICE Bernard Heinrich, MD
5 Garton Road
Rondebosch 7700
Tel. 27-21-683-6544/5 27-21-683-6549
SOUTH AFRICA
Email: bprice@mweb.co.za

RITCHIE Brian, MD
PO Box 11016
Southernwood
Tel. 27-43-726-0566 / 27-43-726-3661
East London, EC 5213
Email: brianrit@telkomsa.net
SOUTH AFRICA

ROBERTSON Joan Leslie Anne, MD
PO Box 70038
Tel. 27-11-463-2268 / 27-11-706-5723
Bryanston 2021
Email: robjla@global.co.za
SOUTH AFRICA

ROBSON Rodney Winston, MD
Morningside Clinic
PO Box 651172
Tel. 27-11-8846165 / 27-11-8833450
Benmore 2010
Email: rodmar@mweb.co.za

Gauteng 2010
SOUTH AFRICA

ROUSSEAU Theodore E., MD
311 Fountain Medical Centre
Heerengracht 8001
Tel. 27-21-421-6069 / 27-21-418-1849
SOUTH AFRICA
Email: ptheos@iafrica.com

SCOTT Peter Desmond, MD
PO Box 651865
Benmore, 2010
Tel. 27-11-883-2135 / 27-11-883-2336
SOUTH AFRICA
Email: peters@cinet.co.za

VAN DER WESTHUIZEN Deon, MD
Cape Town Medi-Clinic
Suite 4006
Tel. 27-21-423-6094 / 27-21-423-7341
21 Hof Street, Gardens 8001
Email: drvdwest@mweb.co.za
147 Green Point 8051
SOUTH AFRICA

VAN WINGERDEN Jan Jouke, MD
Plastic, Reconstructive and Hand Surgery
Medisch Centrum Leeuwarden
Tel. 31-58-28-66-145 / 31-58-28-66-133
PO Box 888
Email: jjvanwingerden@znb.nl
Leeuwarden BR 8901
SOUTH AFRICA

WALTON Russell John, MD
PO Box 751169
Gardenview, 2047
Tel. 27-11-640-1573 / 27-11-640-1579
Johannesburg
Email: drwalton@iafrica.com

SOUTH AFRICA

The South African Medical Association
Block F Castle Walk Corporate Park
Nossob Street
Erasmuskloof X3
POSTAL ADDRESS:
P O Box 74789
Lynnwood Ridge
Pretoria 0040
Tel. (012) 481-2000
Toll free: 0800 110 256
Email: online@samedical.org
http://www.plasticsurgeons.co.za./

Venezuelan Society of Plastic, Reconstructive, Aesthetic and Maxilofacial Surgery
Email: svcprem@cantv.net
(0212)979.73.80
(0212)978.38.86

SOCIETY MEMBERS IN CARACAS
ACQUATELLA, MÁXIME
Centro Médico de Caracas, Anexo A, Piso 1, Cons. 177, San Bernardino.
Telf. 551-19-71, 555- 91- 77
Fax: 576- 72- 61
Celular: 0416-631-08-84

ALAMANOS, ROBERTO
Centro Salud Caracas, Piso 7, Cons. 706, Av. Sorocaima, San Bernardino.
Telefax:550-01-54
Celular: 0414- 320- 24- 13

ALEMÁN MATA, JESÚS
Clínica Venezuela, PB, Cons. 5- A, Alcabala a Peligro N° 7, La Candelaria.
Telf. 573- 38- 32
Fax: 576- 41- 65
BP: 731-51-11/ 07-11 Clave: 9536
Celular: 0414- 281- 57- 43
Email: jesusaleman@terra.com.ve

ALFARO GARANTÓN, JESÚS
Policlínica Santiago de León, Ed. Angostura, Piso 8, Cons. 8-A, Av. Libertador.
Tel.: 762-11-82   Fax: 693-62-17
Celular: 0414-307-21-36
Email: alfagar@cantv.net

ARÉVALO, GUSTAVO
Torre Alfa, Cons. M-2, Av. Principal, Urb. Santa Sofía.
Tel.: 985-45-12 / 02-31
Fax: 985-57-51
Celular: 014-331.33.51

Email: magu11@cantv.net

AYBAR, CARLOS
Torre Hexágono, Piso 4, Av. Rómulo Gallegos, El Marqués. Al lado del Hotel El Marqués.
Tel.: 242- 02- 61 / 02- 81
Fax: 241-16-94
Celular: 0416-622-00- 56
Email: khalilaybar@cantv.net

BARRETO, FELIPE
Instituto de Clínicas y Urología Tamanaco, Cons. 5, PB, San Román.
Tel.: 992- 83- 13 / 99- 10
Telefax: 992- 83- 13
BP:745-11-11 Clave. 6711
Celular: 0416-609-21-55
E- mail: fbm1@telcel.net.ve

BARROS, MARY MIMOSA
Clínica Avila, Piso 10, Cons. 1012, Av. San Juan Bosco, Altamira.
Tel.: 276-10-8 2
Fax: 242-87-74
Celular: 0416-630.06.26
Email: nowacka@cantv.net

BENHAMU, JACK ISAAC
Centro Clínico Profesional Caracas, Cons. Mezz. 1 y 2, Av. Panteón, San Bernardino.
Tel.: 576-01-06/ 37- 94   Fax: 576-37-94
BP:731-51-11/ 07-11 Clave 4061
Celular: 0414-321.48.78
E- mail: benhamuplastic@cantv.net benhamuplastic@guia-medica.com

BRACHO, CARLOS
Centro Salud Caracas, Piso 6, Cons. 603, Av. Sorocaima, San Bernardino.
Tel.: 550- 26- 62, 551- 40- 11
Celular: 0414-327-82-47

BRITO, ARGENIS
Clínica Santa Sofía, Cons. 207, Av. Principal Santa Sofía. El Cafetal.

Tel.: 985-69-52 / 62-53/ 42- 33
Fax: 987- 45-60
Celular.: 0416-621- 59- 18

BULOZ, JUAN JOSÉ
Ed. Centro Médico Dr. Gaetano Di Bianco, Calle Orinoco con
Mucuchíes, Las Mercedes.
Tel.: 993- 82- 17/ 991- 95-03/ 66- 78
Fax: 991-96-08
Celular: 0416-625- 05- 41

CARDOZO DA SILVA, ANTONIO
Centro Caracas, Piso 7, Cons. 7D, Av. Panteón,
San Bernardino.
Tel.: 577-13- 25/ 14- 95
Fax: 286-34-15 BP: 731-51-11/ 07-11 Clave 23772
Celular: 0416-623-28-49
Email: ajcardozo@cantv.net

CARLESSO, JORGE
Clínica Sanatrix, Piso 1, 4ta. Avenida, Campo Alegre.
Tel.: 265-96-40
Fax: 264-15-86
BP: 731-51-11/ 07- 11 Clave 118
Celular:0414-323-01-47
Email: jcarlessob@etheron.net

CASANOVA, RAFAEL
Centro Clínico Profesional Caracas, Piso 11, Cons. 1112, Av. Panteón,
San Bernardino.
Tel.: 574-25-27, 508-65-43/24-25
Fax: 574-24-05
BP: 267-45-33 Clave 3029
Celular: 0414-324-76-65
Email: cas338@telcel.net.ve

CASTILLO ROJAS, CARLOS
Clínica Sanatrix, 4ta.Avenida, Campo Alegre.
Tel.: 265-96-40/ 201- 21-04
Celular: 0414-235-21-16
Email: cecerre3@cantv.net

CASTRO GARCÍA, JORGE
Clínica Sanatrix, Piso 1, Cons. 101, 4ta. Avenida, Campo Alegre.
Tel.: 267-30-22 / 21-06 Ext. 101
Fax: 263-88-07
Celular:0412-277-29-22
Email: jcastrog@telcel.net.ve

CEBALLOS, LUIS
Calle Centro No. 127, Qta. Girasol, Urb. Santa Sofía.
Hab/Fax: 987-14-31
Celular: 0416-828-06-76
Email: marbellal@cantv.net

CEMBORAÍN, MARISELA
Centro Clínico Profesional Caracas, Piso 11, Cons. 11-11, Av. Panteón,
San Bernardino.
Tel.: 578-21-11/16-94, 945-83-35, 949-62-92
Fax: 693-68-59
BP: 731-51-11/ 07-11 Clave 0402
Celular: 0414-321.37-64
Email: mcemborain@cantv.net

CHACON CASTRO, CESAR
Policlínica La Arboleda, PB, Cons. 7, Av. Cajigal, San Bernardino.
Tel.: 551-70-04 Ext. 307
Celular: 0414-314-79-79
Email: ceaugus@telcel.net

CHANG, ROGER
Clínica Vista Alegre, Cons. 6, Calle 3, Vista Alegre. Tel.: 471- 70-18

Celular: 0414-274-56-22

CHIRINOS, MIGUEL ANGEL
Centro Caracas, Piso 4, Cons. 4-B, Final Av. Panteón, San Bernardino.
Tel.: 576-90-60 / 90-39/ 90-71
Fax: 570-90-51
Celular: 0416-622-18-46
Email: chirinos4@hotmail.com

COELLO, ALFREDO
Clínica El Ávila, Piso 10 Cons. 1007, Altamira.
Telefax.: 662-64-92, 262-04-04
BP: 731-51-11/07-11 Clave 983
Celular: 0416-622-65-80
Email: acoello2@hotmail.com

CONTARIS, ANGEL
Clínica Jaimes Córdova, Cons. 2, Av. Simón Planas, Santa Mónica.
Tel.: 662-60-06, 662-86-87
Fax: 662-54-12
Celular: 0412-576-12-14

CONTASTI, RAFAEL
Clínica Vista Alegre, Calle 3, Vista Alegre.
Tel.: 472-97-47
Telefax: 471-37-54
Unidad Clínica Quirúrgica Santa Rosa de Lima. Tel.: 993-10-42
BP: 800- BUSCA Clave 31874
Celular: 0414-321-41-63
Email: miraf@cantv.net

CORZO, EVELIO
Torre Maracaibo, Piso 5, Consultorio 5-B, Av. Libertador.
Tel.: 762-16-17
Celular: 0416-623-25-20
Email: ecorzos@hotmail.com

DELGADO ARISTIMUÑO, CARMEN
Clínica Las Ciencias, Cons. 4, Calle Los Abogados, Los Chaguaramos.
Tel.: 661-67-62, 662-96-80
Celular: 0416-622-21-04

DE ABAFFY STEFFENS, ANNA MARIA
Celular: 0414-323-35-84
Email: anamatito@hotmail.com

DE ALMEIDA, CORALIA
Celular: 0414-332-12-84
DE SOUSA, ALEXIS
Instituto Diagnóstico, Anexo 1, Cons. 302, Av. Anauco, San Bernardino.

Tel.: 552-62-37, 551-11-33
Fax: 963-51-83
Celular: 0416-622-03-36
Email: adesousa@cantv.net

DE VALDÉS, FERNANDO
Clínica Dr. Fernando de Valdés, Calle California, Qta. Carmelina, Las Mercedes.
Tel.: 993-49-34
Telefax: 993.55-58
Celular: 0414-329-36-29
Email: ferval@telcel.net

DEL BIANCO BRUNO (Titular)
Policlínica Méndez Gimón, Cons. 2, Av. Andrés Bello, Las Palmas.
Tel.: 782-04-21
Fax: 662-64-92, 782-36-39
Celular: 0416-622-65-81

DEL REGUERO, ANTONIO (Titular)
Centro Médico de Caracas, Anexo A, Sótano 1, Cons. 18, San Bernardino.
Tel.: 552-59-19, 551-70-76
Celular: 0414-327-12-47
Email: adelre@cantv.net

DÍAZ PORTOCARRERO, JESÚS (Titular)
Centro Médico de Caracas, Anexo C (Medicentro), Piso 1, Cons. 1-D, San Bernardino.
Tel.: 552-80-09 / 46-86
Fax: 552-54-27
BP: 731-51-11/ 07-11 Clave 1024
Email: chudiaz@hotmail.com

DOW, GARIB
Clínica Santa Sofía, Piso 1, Cons. 109, Av. Principal, Urb. Santa Sofía.
Tel.: 985-41-22, 981-11-09
Instituto Urológico San Román, Sector San Román, Las Mercedes.
Telefax: 991-52-42/ 57-31
Celular: 0414-321-69-79

Email: gadow@telcel.net.ve

ESCOBAR RODRÍGUEZ, IGNACIO
Centro Profesional Oeste, Callejón Machado,
Piso 3, Cons. 31, El Paraíso.
Tel.: 483-42-45
Celular:0414-324-49-98
Email: ignacioescobar@cantv.net

FARIÑAS, NICOMEDES (Titular)
Hospital de Clínicas Caracas, Sótano 1, Cons. 2, Av. Panteón, San
Bernardino.
Tel.: 574-08-24 / 99-16
Fax: 406-12-18
BP: 731-51-11/ 07-11 Clave 116
Celular: 0416-620-78-50
Email: nfarinasg@hotmail.com

FERNÁNDES ANDRADE, JUAN SERGIO
Clínica Vista Alegre. Anexo Cons. 21. 3ra Calle, Urb. Vista Alegre.
Tel.: 471-36-28   Fax: 472-77-24
Celular: 0416-630-62-87
Email: juanimaru@cantv.net

FERNÁNDEZ PEÑUELA, RANDOLFO
Celular: 0414-313-61-59
Email: ranfolfo@cantv.net
          rfernandez@guia-medica.com

FÍGALLO ELEAZAR (Titular)
Clínica El Avila, Piso 9, Cons. 910-911, Av. San Juan Bosco, Altamira.
Tel.: 261-43-71
Telefax: 261-15-55
Email: efigallo@clinicaelavila.com

FÍGALLO, ROSARIO
Clínica Sanatrix, Cons. 208, 4ta. Transversal, Campo Alegre.
Tel.: 201-22-28, 267-30-22/ 19-08
Celular: 0416-631-26-44
Fax: 201-21-22

Email: joch3@supercable.net.ve

FLICKI, ENRIQUE
Hospital de Clínicas Caracas, Cons. 315, San Bernardino.
Tel.: 574-53-53
BP: 731-51-11/ 07-11 Clave 2808
Email: eflicky@cantv.net

FLORES, DALIA
Unidad Oftalmológica González Sirit, Av. Luis
Roche con 6a Transversal, Altamira.
Telefax.: 285-35-88/ 43-87, 286-87-33
Celular: 0416-621-75-43
Email: gonzalezsirit@cantv.net

FOUQUET QUIÑONES, AIDA
Centro Médico Quirúrgico San Antonio. Centro Comercial Galería Las
Americas. Nivel Mezz. San Antonio de los Altos.
Tel.: 373 –61- 20/ 60- 75
Centro Clínico de la Policía Metropolitana. San
Martín.
Tel.: 451-11-39
Celular: 0412-739-37-15

FUENMAYOR, GERMAN (Titular)
Clínica Leopoldo Aguerrevere, Piso 2, Cons.
205, Calle Río, Parque Humboldt.
Telefax: 979-23-75/ 71-79
Celular:
Email: fuenma@telcel.net.ve
        gfuenm@hotmail.com

GALINDO ECHEANDIA, ROGER
Instituto de Cirugía Plástica, Av. Tocuyo, Colinas de Bello Monte,
Caracas 1050.
Tel.: 751-86-97   Fax: 751-96-08
Celular: 0416-630-13-71
Email: rogergalindo@yahoo.com

GALINDO TRIAS, ROGER (Titular)

Clínica Santa Sofía, Cons. 203, Av. Principal Santa Sofía.
Tel.: 985-68-72
Fax: 985-76-01
Instituto de Cirugía Integral, Colinas de Bello Monte.
Tel.: 751-37-28 / 86-97
Fax: 751-96-08
Celular: 0416-624-69-80
Email: plastika@telcel.net.ve

GARCÍA DEL MORAL, MARGARITA
Hospital Vargas, servicio de Cirugía Plástica, San José, Caracas.
Centro Ortopédico y Podología, Piso 3, Av. Los Erasos, San Bernardino.
Tel.: 551-28-79
Celular: 0414-905-64-46
Email: gamo@etheron.net

GARRIDO, ZAIDA
Centro Clínico La Urbina, Cons. 13, Calle 6 con calle 7, La Urbina.
Tel.: 241-57-60 / 30-89
Celular: 0416-625-93-75

GARROZ, CORINA
Clínica Luis Razetti, Piso 1, Cons. 33, Av. Este 2. Bellas Artes.
Tel.: 572-87-41 – 597-03-33
Celular: 0412-715-69-29

GIL, ORLANDO
Clínica Caurimare, Cons. 25, Anexo A, Av. Caurimare, Bello Monte.
Tel.: 754-06-25
Telefax: 751-18-66
Celular: 0414-218-90-45

GIMÉNEZ, ZAIDETH
Clínica CEMO, Av. Arturo Michelena entre Reinaldo Hans y Simón
Planas, Consultorio 207. Santa Mónica.
Tel.: 693-48-29 ext. 117.
Celular: 0416-627-21-68

GIULIANO D'ANGELO, SEBASTIÁN
Instituto Clínico La Florida, Piso 2, Cons. 13, Av. Los Samanes, La
Florida.

Tel.: 706-60-14 / 60-21
Fax: 730-92-54
BP: 761-21-11 Clave 1677
Celular: 0416-623-56-37

GONCALVES, ANTONIO
Instituto Clínico La Florida, Area D, Cons. 6-8, Av. Los Samanes, La
Florida.
Tel.: 706- 61-24 Telefax: 706-61-46
Celular: 0414-322-39-96
Email: agoncalvesfdr@msn.com

GONCALVES, JOSÉ CARLOS
Clínica Vista Alegre, Cons. 27, PB, Calle 3, Vista Alegre.
Tel.: 471-11-47
BP: 800- BUSCA Clave 9647
Celular: 0414-321-41-93
Email: cardocto@telcel.net.ve

GONZÁLEZ CARLOS LUIS
Policlínica Santiago de León, Ed. Angostura, Piso 6, Cons. 6-B, Av.
Libertador.
Tel.: 763-54-76   Fax: 762-71-83
Celular: 0414-930-63-64
Email: clgs2231@telcel.net.ve

GONZÁLEZ BAQUERIZO, MEDARDO
Centro Clínico Profesional Caracas, Piso 8, Cons.804, Av. Panteón, San
Bernardino.
Tel.: 574-42-45/ 64-79
Fax: 238-37-30
Celular: 0414-322-97-83
Email: 0414-322-97-83@mipunto.com

GORDON PARRA, MANUEL V.
Instituto La Florida, Cons. 10, PB. Av. Los Samanes Norte. La Florida.
Telefax: 706-60-48
Celular: 0414-337-58-06
Email: maniven@cantv.com

GOTTENGER, RAFAEL

Email: rgotten@hotmail.com

GUTIÉRREZ, FRANCISCO
Policlínica Santiago de León, Torre Negrín, Piso 5, Av. Libertador.
Tel.: 762-46-95/ 79-71, 761-45-09
Celular: 0416-623-30-99

GUZMAN, PEDRO
Clínica Razetti, Piso 1, Cons. 33, Av. Este 2, Bellas Artes.
Tel.: 572-87-41, 597-03-33
Fax: 991-26-64
Celular: 0414-327-29-70
E-mail. petete@telcel.net.ve

HENRÍQUEZ, EDMUNDO
Clínica La Floresta, Anexo, Av. Santa Ana, La Floresta.
Tel.: 284-19-22/ 10-63
Fax: 284-07-32
BP: 731.51-11/ 07-11 Clave 1145
Celular: 0416-621-23-49
Email: edmundohenriquez@hotmail.com

HIDALGO, PABLO
Clínica Santa Sofía, Torre Alfa, Mezz. Cons. M-2, Av. Principal Santa Sofía.
Tel.: 985-45-12 / 02-31
Fax: 985-57-51
Celular: 0416-622-49-58
Email: pabloh@unete.com.ve
        pabloh@ifxnw.com.ve
        pablohidalgo@yahoo.com

HOLLEBECQ, ANA
Centro Médico Quirúrgico del Sur, Calle Rufino Blanco Fombona, Santa Mónica.
Telefax.: 662-64-92, 262-04-04
BP: 731-51-11/ 07-11 Clave 496
Celular: 0416-627-45-40
Email: acoello2@hotmail.com

KAAKEDJIAN, GARBIS

Policlínica Metropolitana, Piso 1, Cons. 132, Calle A-1, Caurimare.
Tel.: 908-06-36, 985-71-41
BP: 267-45-33 Clave 1809
Celular: 0414-325-70-88
Email: kaakedjiangarbis@hotmail.com

KUBE, REINALDO
Clínica El Avila, Cons. 812, Altamira.
Tel.: 276-18-82 / 18-83
Fax: 274-09-69
BP: 267-45-33 Clave 3429
Celular: 0414-325-76-47   0412-325-76-47
Email: reiaid@cantv.net

LAU PÉREZ, MAGDALENA CRISTINA
Grupo de Especialistas Washington, Cons. 2, Av. Washington, El
Paraíso.
Tel.: 461-14-42 / 73-80 / 59-56
Centro Médico Quirúrgico VidaMed
Av. Francisco Solano López con Calle El Cristo, Piso 4. Cons. 401.
Sabana Grande. El Recreo.
Tel.: 762-3098/ 761-0799/ 761-6009
Celular: 0416-614-03-13
Email: malelaup@hotmail.com

MANRIQUE, MARÍA CAROLINA
Clínica Luis Razetti, Piso 1, Cons. 41, Av. Este 2, Bellas Artes.
Tel.: 575-06-48, 597-03-46, 574-86-46/ 02-57
Celular: 0414-312-36-08
Email: mcmanrique@telcel.net.ve

MARCANO DE CUENCA, ROSA T.
Hospital Universitario de Caracas, Unidad de Cirugía Plástica. Sótano.
Tel.: 606-73-15
Celular: 0414-322-92-40
Email: rmcuenca@telcel.net.ve

MÁRQUEZ, CLAUDIO
Instituto Clínico La Florida, Calle Los Samanes, La Florida.
Tel.: 706-60.32

MARTELO DE FLORIK, MARÍA DEL
Multicentro Empresarial del Este, Torre Libertador, Núcleo B, Piso 7, Cons. 71-B, Chacao.
Tel.: 263-70-30 / 70-10
Fax: 263 68 56
Email: russoflorik@cantv.net

MARTÍNEZ, EDGAR
Centro de Cirugía Ambulatoria Solano, Ofic. Norte, Ed. Torre Banco Andino, Esq. Los Jabillos, Av. Francisco Solano.
Tel.: 762-47-97 / 47-96
Fax: 762-56-52
Celular: 0416-625-73-39
Email: martinezedgar@cantv.net

MARTÍNEZ DE LA RIVA, PATRICIA
Policlínica Metropolitana, Piso 2, Cons. 2-34, Calle A-1, Caurimare.
Tel.: 908-06-45, 987-45-23
Fax: 985-97-41
BP: 952-86-44 Clave 0319
Celular: 0414-408-89-61

MAYORCA, EDUARDO
Clínica San Pablo, Calle La Peña y La Guairita, Las Mercedes.
Tel.: 992-07-93 / 22-11
Fax: 234-56-05

BP: 731-51-11/ 07-11 Clave 4016
Celular: 0414-921-11-91
Email: educrisma@telcel.net.ve

MENESES IMBER, PEDRO
C.I: 5.305.928.
Hospital de Clínicas Caracas, Cons. 308, San Bernardino.
Tel.: 508-63-08, 576-69-66
Fax: 731-72-68
BP: 731-51-11/ 07-11 Clave 2643
Celular: 0414-931-77-88
Email: pmeneses@hotmail.com

MÍGUEZ NOVOA, JOSEFINA
C.I: 5.607.941.
Centro Clínico Profesional Caracas, Piso 6, Cons. 6-06, Av. Panteón, San Bernardino.
Tel.: 574-65-27/ 54-27
Fax: 574-16-94
Celular: 0416-622-76-38
Email: jmiguezn@cantv.net

MOGOLLÓN, EVELIN
Centro de Especialidades Médicas, UNISAES, Final Av. Madrid # 21-38, La California Norte.
Tel.: 271-60-71, 272-03-02
Fax: 272- 21-90
Celular: 0414-251-18-04

MONTICELLI, DIANA
Policlínica Metropolitana, Piso 2, Cons. 232-234, Calle A-1, Caurimare.
Tel.: 908-06-45 / 06-79   Fax: 985-97-41
BP: 952-86-44 Clave 5820317
Celular: 0416-630-02-04
Email: galuppo-ve@yahoo.com

MONTILLA VELÁSQUEZ, JOSE F.
Hospital Militar "Dr. Carlos Arvelo".
Tel.: 406-15.55 / 11-56/ 11-11
Fax: 681-63-57
Celular: 0416-620-42-94
BP: 731-51 -11/ 07-11 Clave 1328

MORALES, TRINA
Policlínica Méndez Gimón, Piso 3, Cons. 20, Av. Andrés Bello, Las Palmas.
Tel.: 793-27-36
Celular: 0416-609- 05-15
Email: muljca@telcel.net.ve

MORALES BELLO, DAVID
Centro Comercial Macaracuay Plaza, Torre B, Piso 7. CIME.

Tel.: 257-39-98/ 39-23
Celular:0416-639-48-01
Email: dmoralesbello@cantv.net

NARCISO, LUIS ALBERTO
Policlínica Metropolitana, Piso 2, Cons. 2-0, Calle A-1, Caurimare.
Tel.: 908-02-64 / 02-65 / 01-00
Fax: 963.71.33
Celular: 0416-633-73-73

NARCISO CHACÓN, MARISELA
Policlínica Metropolitana, Piso 2, Cons. 2-0, Calle A-1, Caurimare.
Tel.: 908-02-64 / 02-65 / 01-00
Fax: 963-71-33
Celular: 0416-615-78-58
Email: mnarciso@cantv.net

NIETO SÁNCHEZ, CARLOS
Clínica San Pablo, Piso 2, Cons. 215, Calle La Peña con La Guairita, Las Mercedes.
Tel.: 992-47-23, 991-24-29, 993-35-61
Celular: 0416-630-70-11
Email: crnieto@cantv.net

NUSSER KIELWEIN, SIMONE
Ambulatorio MEDIS. Centro Comercial Santa Fe.
Tel.: 975-03-29/ 01-40
Fax: 976-64-17
Celular: 0412-234-18-85
E-mail.: simonenusser@cantv.net

OCHOA S., JOSÉ FRANCISCO
Centro Médico de Caracas, Anexo A, Piso 3, Cons. 377, San Bernardino.
Tel.: 552-04-24, 555-93-77
BP: 731-51-11/ 07-11 Clave 01495
Celular: 0412-624-62-53
Email: ochoaneri@cantv.net

ODERIZ, ANTONIO
Hospital Clínico Universitario, Unidad de Cirugía Plástica. Sótano.
Tel.: 606-73-15

OJEDA, FRANCISCO
Unidad de Cirugía Plástica, Calle California entre Monterrey y Mucuchíes,
Qta. Carmelina, Las Mercedes.
Tel.: 993- 55-58/ 49-34
Fax: 993-55-88
Celular: 0414-327-12-80
Email: pancho98@telcel.net.ve

OLIVARES RAMÍREZ, JUAN JOSÉ
Centro Clínico Profesional Caracas, Piso 6, Cons. 614, Av. Panteón, San
Bernardino.
Tel.: 577-43-61   Fax: 576-80-20
Celular: 0416-622-71-34
Email: jjolivares@cantv.net

ONORATO BARRA, MARIO
Instituto Clínico La Florida, Área E, Cons. G, Calle Los Samanes, La
Florida.
Tel.: 706-61-22
Celular: 0414-288-62-38
Email: moplastico@telcel.net.ve

ORTEGA LARA, JOSÉ
Policlínica Méndez Gimón, Cons. 12-A, Av. Andrés Bello, Las Palmas.
Tel.: 793- 61-81   Fax: 793-21-07
Celular:0414-325-34-77
Email: jortegal@cantv.net

OZIEL, MARCOS
Clínica La Floresta, Cons. 122, Calle Santa Ana, La Floresta.
Tel.: 209-61-32   Fax: 286-17-10
Celular: 0416-627-49-30
Email: marcooozielzz@hotmail.com

PÁRRAGA DE Z. BETTY
Clínica El Avila, Piso 10, Cons. 1004, Av. San Juan Bosco, Altamira.
Tel.: 261-37-68   Fax: 261-55-40
BP: 731-51-11/ 07-11 Clave 552
Celular: 0416-621-91-40
Email: betty_zoghbi@hotmail.com

PEÑA, ÁNGEL
Centro Comercial Sta. Fe, Nivel Valle Arriba, Local C-3, Sta. Fe.
Tel.: 976-16-93 al 96 Ext. 124
Celular: 0412-378-38-45
Email: alabamaleo91@telcel.net.ve

PEREIRA MALDONADO, JESÚS O.
Centro Comercial Lido, Nivel Galeria, Local GH, Chacaito
Tel.: 550-26-62   Fax: 574-58-64
Celular: 0414-320-43-31
Email: jorpem@telcel.net.ve

PÉREZ MORELL, ALBERTO
Instituto Médico La Floresta, PB. Cons. 704, Av. Principal de la Floresta
con Calle Sta. Ana.
Tel.: 209-62-22 Ext. 618
Telefax: 284- 55- 23
BP: 731-51-11/ 07-11 Clave 5246
Celular: 0416-633-42-04
Email: albertyale@hotmail.com

PETIT PIFANO, GUIDO (Titular)
Centro Médico de Caracas, Anexo A, Cons. 76, San Bernardino.
Tel.: 552-04-04, 509-91-66
Fax: 552-03-75
Celular: 0416-622-00-55
Email: gpetita@etheron.net

PIERINI, MARÍA ROSA
Clínica Loira. Piso 7, Cons.701, Urb. Loira.
El Paraíso.
Tel.: 405-21-51
Celular: 0414-245-33-65
PIÑERÚA, SONIA
Policlínica Metropolitana, Piso 2, Cons. 2-0, Calle A-1, Caurimare.
Tel.: 908.02.64/ 02-65, 986-41-21
Celular: 0414-209-82-73

POCOROBA ARA, ALEJANDRO
Centro Perú, Torre B, Piso 9, Cons. 94, Chacao.

Tel.: 266-13-25
Fax: 266-01-62
BP: 731-51-11/ 07-11 Clave 13997
Celular: 0416-639-95-13

POLANCO, FABIO
Policlínica Santiago de León, Torre Maracaibo, Piso 14, Cons. B, Av. Libertador.
Tel.: 763-45-18, 508-43-15
Email: fabiopolanco@hotmail.com

PONCE, MARIO
Policlínica Metropolitana, Cons. 3-L, Calle A-1, Caurimare.
Tel.: 908-03-60, 985-75-76
Fax: 985-22-69
BP: 952-86-44 Clave 0318
Celular: 0416-624-24-67
Email: mario@rapidnet.net.ve

POZO, HILDA
Policlínica Americana, Cons. 3C, Av. Venezuela, El Rosal.
Telefax.: 952-53-37
Celular: 0416-623-39-98
Email: lacastro@reacciun.ve

QUISPE MORALES, MARIO
Centro de Cirugía Estética TUMI, Torre Profesional, Piso 9, Cons. 17, Centro Comercial Palo Verde, Petare.
Tel.: 251-31-76
Celular: 0416-715-09-91

RADA, VÍCTOR MANUEL
Centro Clínico Vista California, Calle Trieste, Los Ruices Sur.
Tel.: 256- 46- 22, 257- 00- 11/ 33- 33
Fax: 257- 27- 42/ 953-42-87
Celular: 0416-637-29-97
Email: rada7893@cantv.net

RINCÓN, LINDA LORENA
Centro Clínico Profesional Caracas, Piso 11, Cons. 11-11, Av. Panteón, San Bernardino.

Tel.: 578-21-15/ 25-95
BP: 731-51-11/ 07-11 Clave 9491
Urológico San Román. Cons. W- 2.
Tel.: 999-05-86
Celular: 0414-331-23-79
Email: lindal@cantv.net

RINCÓN DURÁN, NILYAN B.
Centro Clínico Vista California, Calle Trieste, Los Ruices Sur.
Tel.: 256- 46- 22, 257- 00- 11/ 33- 33
Fax: 257- 27- 42
Hospital Oncológico Padre Machado
Tel.: 631-01-36
Celular: 0414-272-94-32
Email: nilian@cantv.net

RINCONES, JOSÉ MANUEL
Centro Clínico Profesional Caracas, Piso 12, Cons. 1212, San
Bernardino.
Tel.: 577-15-77   Fax: 975-53-95
Celular: 0414-930-78-99
Email: jrincone@telcel.net.ve

RODRÍGUEZ, ALEXIS
Torre Alfa, Piso 7, Cons. 7-C. Av. Ppal. Sta. Sofía. (Frente Clínica Sta.
Sofía).
Tel.: 985-43-15
Instituto de Cirugía Plástica, Av. El Tocuyo, Colinas de Bello Monte.
Tel.: 751-37-28 / 86-97
Fax: 751-96-08
Celular: 0416-624-07-38
Email: plastika@telcel.net.ve

RODRÍGUEZ, BLANCA
Instituto de Medicina Integral. Piso 3, Cons. 3-N, Av. Mariscal Sucre,
San Bernardino.
Tel.: 552-23-93
Fax: 550-04-12
Celular: 0416-608-69-17

RODRÍGUEZ, FRANCISCO

Policlínica Metropolitana, Cons. 132, Calle
A-1, Caurimare.
Tel.: 987-35-45, 908-06-36
Fax: 753-87-38
BP: 731-51-11/ 07-11 Clave 4074
Celular:0414-306-44-66

RODRÍGUEZ, ISMAEL
Centro Caracas, Piso 4, Cons. 4B, Av. Panteón con Av. Los Erasos, San
Bernardino.
Tel.: 576-90-60/ 90-39
Fax: 570-90-51
Celular: 0414-209-02-32

RODRÍGUEZ, NELSON
Instituto Médico La Floresta, Cons. 216, Calle Santa Ana, La Floresta.
Telefax.: 284-65-65, 209-62-22
BP: 731-51-11/ 07-11 Clave 2962
Celular: 0412-722-41-09

RODRÍGUEZ P., PEDRO
Policlínica El Paraíso, Consultorio # 3, Av. Washington # 33, El
Paraíso.
Tel.: 461-29-57
Celular: 0416-637-54-54
Email: rodriguezcurcio@cantv.net

RODRÍGUEZ, RAÚL
Centro Clínico Profesional Caracas, Piso 3, Cons. 3-09, Av. Panteón,
San Bernardino.
Telefax.: 577-77-03
BP: 761-21-11 Clave 1934
Celular: 0416-625-77-01

RÖMER PIERETTI, PETER
Clínica La Floresta, Piso 2, Cons. 211, Calle Santa Ana, La
Floresta.
Tel.: 284-19-22/ 10-63, 209-62-22
Fax: 977-40-21
Celular: 0414-920-06-97
Email: pvromer@unete.com.ve

RUSSO, SALOMÓN
Multicentro Empresarial del Este, Torre Libertador. Núcleo B, Piso 7,
Cons. 71-B, Chacao.
Tel.: 263-70-30 / 70-10   Fax: 263-68-56
Celular: 0414-320-48-28
Email: russoflorik@cantv.net

SABOÍN, JOSÉ LUIS
Centro Clínico Profesional Caracas, Piso 4, Cons. 411, Av. Panteón . San
Bernardino.
Tel.: 574-96-68/ 45-78
Celular: 0416-624-30-73

SANOJA,   RAMÓN
Centro de Especialidades Médicas, UNISAES, Final Av. Madrid # 21-38,
La California Norte.
Tel.: 271-60-71, 272-03-02
Fax: 272- 21-90
Celular: 0414-244-84-05
Email: sanojao@cantv.net

SAUCE,   OSWALDO   (Titular)
Clínica El Ávila, Piso 5, Cons. 511, Av. San Juan Bosco, Altamira.
Tel.:262-20-79/21-79
Fax: 261-18-11
Celular: 0416-622-57-56
Email: osauce@clinicaelavila.com

SERRANO,   JULIO
Policlínica La Arboleda, Cons. 1, Av. Cajigal, San Bernardino.Lun.Mier-
Vier. 3:00pm a 8:00pm
Tel.: 551-66-13/ 65-50/ 18-11 Ext. 301
Fax: 731-28-68
Instituto Médico SERWAL C.A.
Calle el Retiro. Edf. Sandrita PB. N° 1.
Urb . Ávila. Alta Florida.
Tel.: 415-03-77
BP: 731-61-11 Clave 06966

Celular: 0414-325-10-33
Email: julioserrano23@hotmail.com

SIFONTES, GUSTAVO
Instituto Clínico La Florida, PB, Cons. 4, Calle Los Samanes, La Florida.
Tel.: 730-45-66 / 48-75
Celular: 0416-811-98-72

SLOBODIANIK CORREA, DANIEL
Grupo Médico Libertador, Torre Libertador 75, PH- A1, Av. Libertador.
Telefax: 761-82-55/ 30-90
BP: 263-62-11 Clave 1950
Celular: 0414-312-04-78
Email: plastic@surgical.net
        www.cirugiaplastica.com.ve
Fax: 265-36-27
Celular: 0416-622-10-72
Email: beatrizsos@cantv.net

SOUSA GADEA, IGNACIO
Policlínica Metropolitana, Piso 1, Cons. 1-U, Caurimare.
Tel.: 908-03-60, 985-75-76
Fax: 985-22-69
BP: 952-86-44 Clave 5820320
Celular: 0412-624-66-27
Email: ignacio@rapidnet.net.ve

SUÁREZ, GUILLERMO (Titular)
Policlínica Méndez Gimón, Cons. 19, Av. Andrés Bello, Las Palmas.
Tel.: 793-16-22, 794-19-39, 781-68-01
Celular: 0414-920-65-75
Email: henrys@telcel.net.ve

TENAILLE, JEAN
Clínica Caurimare, Anexo A, Cons. 28, Av. Caurimare, Bello Monte.
Tel.: 751-18-63
Celular: 0416-637-80-58

TERIFE, CECILIO
Clínica Razetti, PB, Cons. 14, Av. Este 2 Sur 21, Bellas
Artes.   Tel.: 572-06-92

Apartado Postal 17.192, Parque Central, Caracas 1015-A.
Tel.: 509-22-04 / 22-27
BP: 751-31-11/ 07-11 Clave 21991

THEN, ROSARIO
Clínica Loira, Piso 8, Cons.07,Av. Loira, El Paraíso.

Tel.: 405-23-46/ 21-11, 451-14-15
Celular: 0414-326-85-50

TROCONIS, JOSÉ RAFAEL (Titular)
Instituto de Clínicas y Urología Tamanaco, Cons. 13-A, Calle Chivacoa, San Román.
Tel.: 999-01-59 / 01-58
BP: 731-51-11/ 07-11 Clave 2238
Celular: 0416-623-63-62
Email: jtroconis@reacciun.ve

URDANETA, CARMEN
Centro Clínico, Cons. 22, Calle Tito Salas entre Av. México y Esquina Colimodio, La Candelaria.
Tel.: 572-88-58
Fax: 731-58-32
Celular: 0414-205-98-91

VALENTE, LUCIO
Clínica El Ávila, Piso 8, Cons. 808, Av. San Juan Bosco, Altamira.
Tel.: 276-18-68, 263-00-56
Fax: 276-18-59, 264-54-76
Celular: 0414-205-98-91
Email: office@luciovalente.com
         www.luciovalente.com

VÁSQUEZ, EDGAR
Policlínica Metropolitana, Piso 1, Cons. 1-38, Calle A-1, Caurimare.
Tel.: 908-06-33 / 01-00
Telefax: 987-24-64
Celular: 0416-622-72-28
Email: pitocom@cantv.net

VEGA, BERNARDO

Instituto Clínico La Florida, Área C, Cons. 6, Calle Los Samanes, La Florida.
Tel.: 706-61-34 / 60-76
BP: 731-51-11/ 07-11 Clave 7740
Celular: 0416-635-82-75

VELÁSQUEZ, IBRAHIM (Titular)
Instituto Diagnóstico, Piso 2, Cons. 21, Av. Anauco, San Bernardino.
Tel.: 555-12-67, 552-40-26
Email: gloriaalidadan@cantv.net

VENTURA, MAIRA
Instituto de Medicina Integral, Piso 3, Cons. 3-N, Av. Mariscal Sucre, San Bernardino.
Tel.: 552-23-93
Fax: 242-97-72
BP: 263-62-11 Clave 1644
Celular: 0414-312-15-01
Email: mairadedascoli@yahoo.com

VILLALOBO GALINDO, GUILLERMO
Torre Alfa, Piso 8, Cons. 8-D. Av. Ppal. Sta. Sofía. (Frente Clínica Sta. Sofía).
Tel.: 985-43-15
 Telefax: 986-43-34
Instituto de Cirugía Plástica, Av. El Tocuyo, Colinas de Bello Monte.
Tel.: 751-37-28/ 86-97
Fax: 751-96-58
Celular: 0416-622-84-93
Email: plastika@telcel.net.ve

VILLAMIZAR MOLINA, ROSABELL
Hospital de Clínicas Oftalmológicas, Av. Louis Braille, Las Acacias.
Tel.: 633-48-10, 632-87-77
Celular: 0412-219-20-00
Email: rosabv@cantv.net

VIZCARRONDO, LEOPOLDO
Policlínica Méndez Gimón, Av. Andrés Bello, PB, Cons. A-2, Las Palmas.

Tel.: 782-04-21
Fax: 782-36-39
Celular: 0416-621-42-44

YASELLI,   DAVID   (Titular)
Centro Profesional Tamanaco, Nivel C-1, Ofic.1, CCCT.
Telefax: 959-69-49/ 73-24
Celular: 0414-317-16-76

YRAUSQUIN, ELIZABETH
Centro Médico de Caracas, Anexo A, Cons. 29, San Bernardino.
Telefax: 552-83-20, 577-72-43
Celular: 0416-615-31-13
Email: elibetty33hotmail.com

ZAPATA SIRVENT, RAMÓN   (Titular)
Centro Médico de Caracas, Anexo A, Piso 1, Cons. 177, San Bernardino.
Tel.: 551-19-71, 55591-77
Fax: 576-72-61
Celular: 0416-624-79-97
Email: zapatasirvent@hotmail.com

Need web site translation?

Go to: http://www.bablefish.altavista.com

Copy the web site URL into the translation box, and change the language to "Spanish to English", then click translate! The translation is not 100% perfect, but you'll get the important stuff!

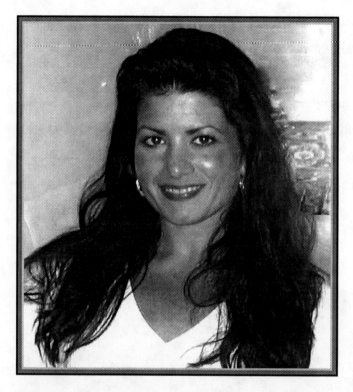

About The Author

JoAnn Roselli is a cosmetic surgery veteran, who has undergone tummy tuck surgery as well as blepharoplasty (eyelid lift), upper arm lift and lipo-sculpture of the upper arms, back, hips, butt and thighs. All her procedures were performed in the Dominican Republic, where she currently lives with her husband and 10-year-old son. She is a former medical transcriptionist, and is currently working as a freelance writer, and unofficial "good will ambassador" for the Dominican Republic. Her spare time is spent painting, writing and "beach hopping" and she is glad you are jealous.

However, she does wish you were here…

Acknowledgements

I would like to thank the following people who assisted me, guided me and encouraged me throughout the process of writing this book: Arturo Moises (my gorgeous research assistant and love of my life), Dr. Roberto Guerrero, Dr. Radhamés Mejia, Dr. Luis E. González Valdez, Guilla V., Amarilis B., the members of http://www.Curzone.com and the MSN Plastic and Cosmetic Surgery Forum, and Mr. Roger Gallo. Works cited in this publication include "Guía Informativa De Cirugía Plastica y Reconstructiva".

RESOURCES

Below you will find Internet addresses where you can find further information and/or purchase products mentioned in the previous text. Simply type the addresses into your web browser window and hit "Go". Be sure to type the URL address exactly as it appears here.

To subscribe to our free newsletter, **"Beautiful on a Budget"**:
http://www.cheap-plastic-surgery.com
or just send a blank email to:
cheapplasticsurgery@getresponse.com

To learn about natural health, parasite cleanse, kidney/bowel/liver cleanses and more, please visit:
http://www.curezone.com

Purchase **"The Cure for All Diseases"** by Dr. Hulda Clark:
http://www.cheap-plastic-surgery.com/clark.html

Cleanse your body and Get Rid of Parasites!
http://www.cheap-plastic-surgery.com/cleanse.html

Get a copy of **"The Artist's Way"** by Julia Cameron:
http://www.cheap-plastic-surgery.com/way.html

Get the Edge with Tony Robbins' help:

http://www.cheap-plastic-surgery.com/tony.html

Read the book **The Sedona Method:**
http://www.cheap-plastic-surgery.com/sedona.html

Centerpointe's Holosync Meditation Personal Growth CDs
http://www.cheap-plastic-surgery.com/holosync.html

Buy Arnica Montana Online
http://www.cheap-plastic-surgery.com/arnica.html

RESOURCES (cont.)

Buy Plastic Surgery Recovery Supplies:
http://www.cheap-plastic-surgery.com/supplies.html

Dr. Laura DiGiorgio's life-changing self-hypnosis**, Stop Smoking, Preparation for Surgery** and **Accelerated Healing After Surgery CDs:**
http://www.cheap-plastic-surgery.com/subliminals.html.

Short-Term Apartment Rentals & Homestays
Services: Short term rentals, homestays, cleaning service, housekeeping, home nursing care, airport transfers, childcare, and more. Apartments and homestays are located in the city of Santo Domingo in the safest and quietest neighborhoods such as Naco, Piantini, El Vergel, Arroyo Hondo, etc.
Email: drinterns@yahoo.com
Phone: 404-270-9182

Casa De Huespedes
Angela Valentin, proprietor
Calle Barbacoa No. 11-A, Cancino 1ro.
Santo Domingo Este, Dominican republic
Tel: (809) 526-7998
Cel: (809) 761-9469

LUXURY PLASTIC SURGERY AND SELF-IMPROVEMENT CARIBBEAN VACATIONS at Affordable Prices!

http://www.cheap-plastic-surgery.com/vacation

For more information via email:

vacation@cheap-plastic-surgery.com

All La Simetria Vacation Packages include:

Luxury private ground transportation to and from the Santo Domingo Airport (SDQ) to as well as all appointments& procedures

7 or 14 day stay in a Beautiful Recovery Suite

Procedure of your choice

One after procedure clinic overnight

24hr Medical after care throughout your stay by a licensed Physician

Personal Assistant on-call

All meals, beverages and snacks

La Simetria Private Label Spring Water

All Non-Alcoholic Beverages

PROCEDURE	Avg. US PROCEDURE ONLY RATE DOES NOT INCLUDE O.R. OR ADDITIONS	La Simetria All-Inclusive Luxury Plastic Surgery Vacation Package	LENGTH OF VACATION
Liposuction	7224 ONE AREA ONLY	6601 MULTIPLE AREAS	14 DAYS
Abdominoplasty	8250	6026	14 DAYS
Buttock Lift	10,000	5451	14 DAYS
Breast Augmentation	8750	6601	14 DAYS
Breast Reduction	7857	5681	14 DAYS
Brachioplasty	6809	5451	14 DAYS
Thighplasty	7823	6026	14 DAYS
Gynecomastia	6939	4163	7 DAYS
Rhinoplasty	7188	4393	7 DAYS
Chin Augmentation	5693	4163	7 DAYS
Otoplasty	6535	4163	7 DAYS
Face Lift	8500	6463	7 DAYS

Airfare is NOT included in Package price yet can be booked and paid for through La Simetria Plastic Surgery Vacation on the airline of your choice.

PAYMENT OPTIONS

We accept Paypal, Visa, MasterCard, AMEX, Wire Transfers, American Express Traveler's Checks and Cash.

FINANCING ALSO AVAILABLE

Information Provided by : ADVANCED PATIENT FINANCING

Example of Monthly Payments Based on 12.99% APR

	60	48	36	24
$2,500	$57	$68	$85	$119
$4,000	$92	$108	$135	$191
$6,000	$137	$162	$203	$286
$10,000	$228	$269	$338	$476
$15,000	$342	$403	$506	$714
$20,000	$456	$538	$675	$952
$25,000	$570	$672	$844	$1192

---------------------* Based on 12.99% APR

How much will your monthly payments be? Simply call Advanced Patient Financing at 1-800-392-5189 and one of their staff members will be pleased to answer your questions, and explain your options to book your La Simetria Plastic Surgery Vacation today!

Patient's FAQ

Q. What if I have credit problems?

A. Advanced Patient Financing has programs for most types of credit histories. If you've been declined in the past by other finance companies, Advanced Patient Financing may still be able to approve your loan request.

Q. What will my interest rate be?

A. Your interest rate is based on your credit history, selected loan term, and loan amount. Patients with excellent credit ratings who apply for financing through Advanced Patient Financing qualify for extra-low interest rates.

Q. Is there a pre-payment penalty?

A. NO! In fact, many of our loans come with a 90-days same as cash feature meaning you actually receive your interest back if you payoff the loan within 90 days.

Q. How do I get more information?

A. One of our staff members will be pleased to answer your questions.

Submit Application at: http://www.cheap-plastic-surgery.com/financing

LaVergne, TN USA
07 February 2010

172329LV00003B/100/A

9 781411 618640